THIS BOOK BELONGS TO :

Emergency Contact Name/Number:

_____

Copyright ©

All rights reserved.
No parts of this publication may be reproduced, distributed, or transmitted in any form, or by any means, including photocopying, recording or other electronic or mechanical methods, without prior written permission from the publisher.

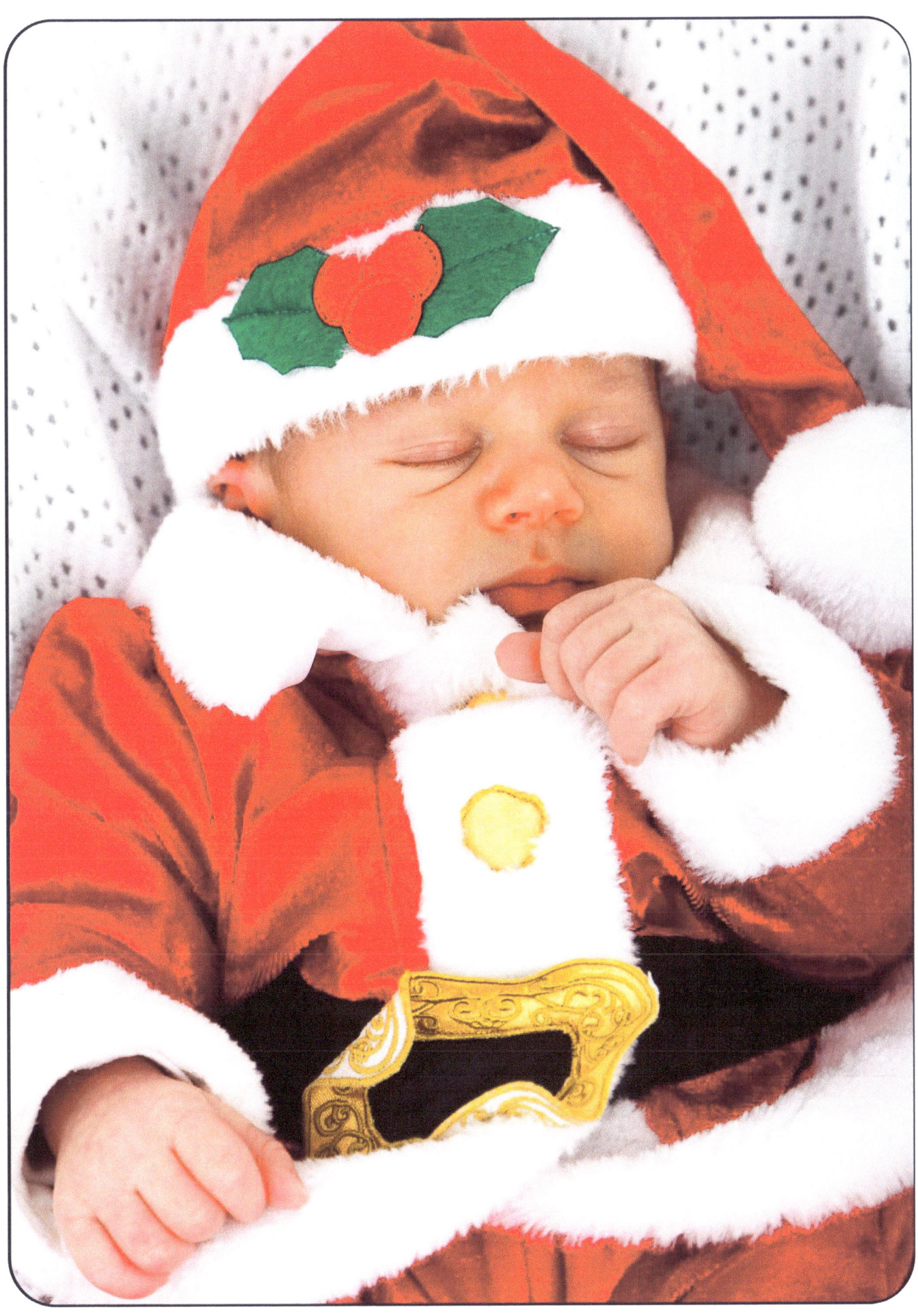

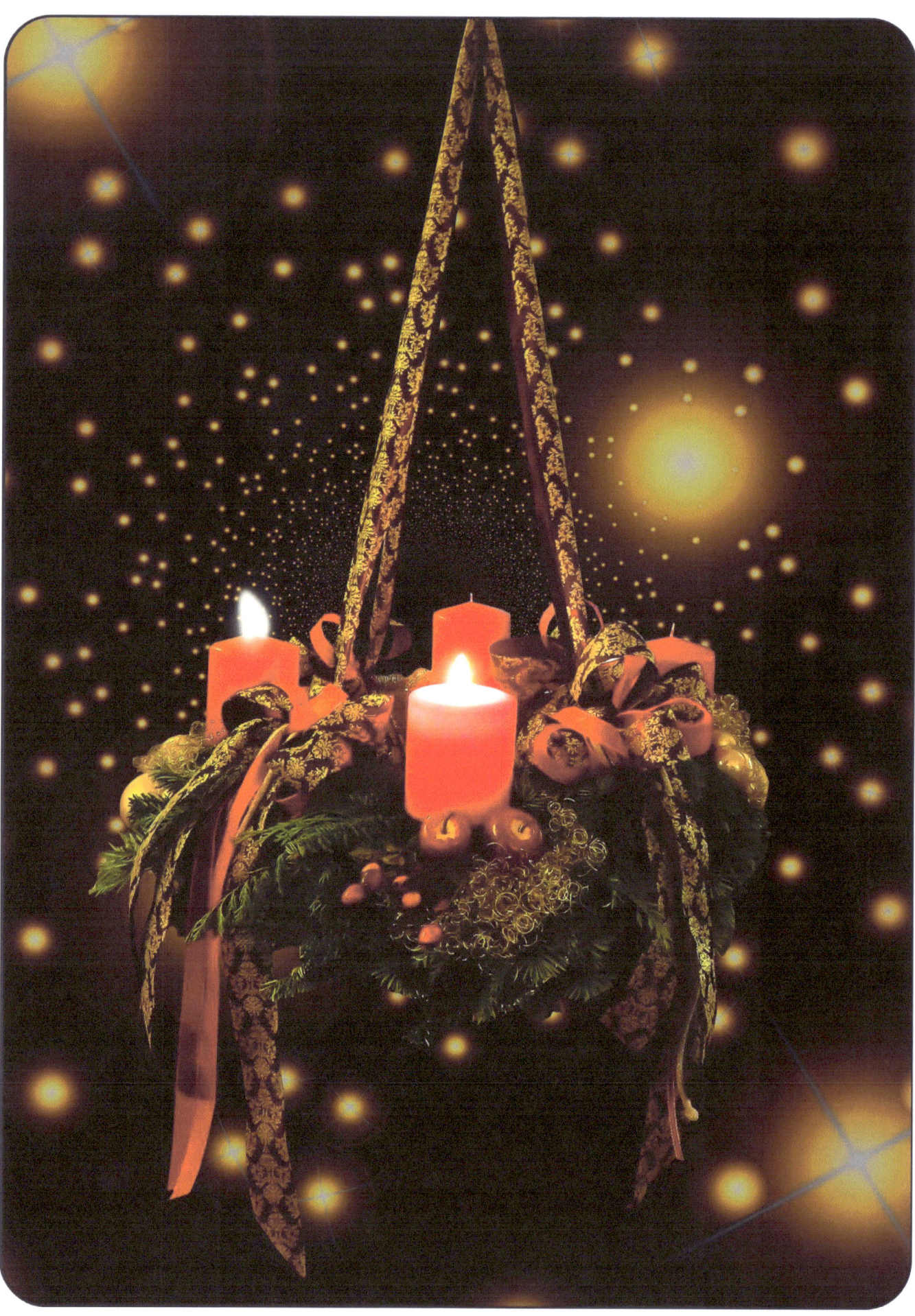

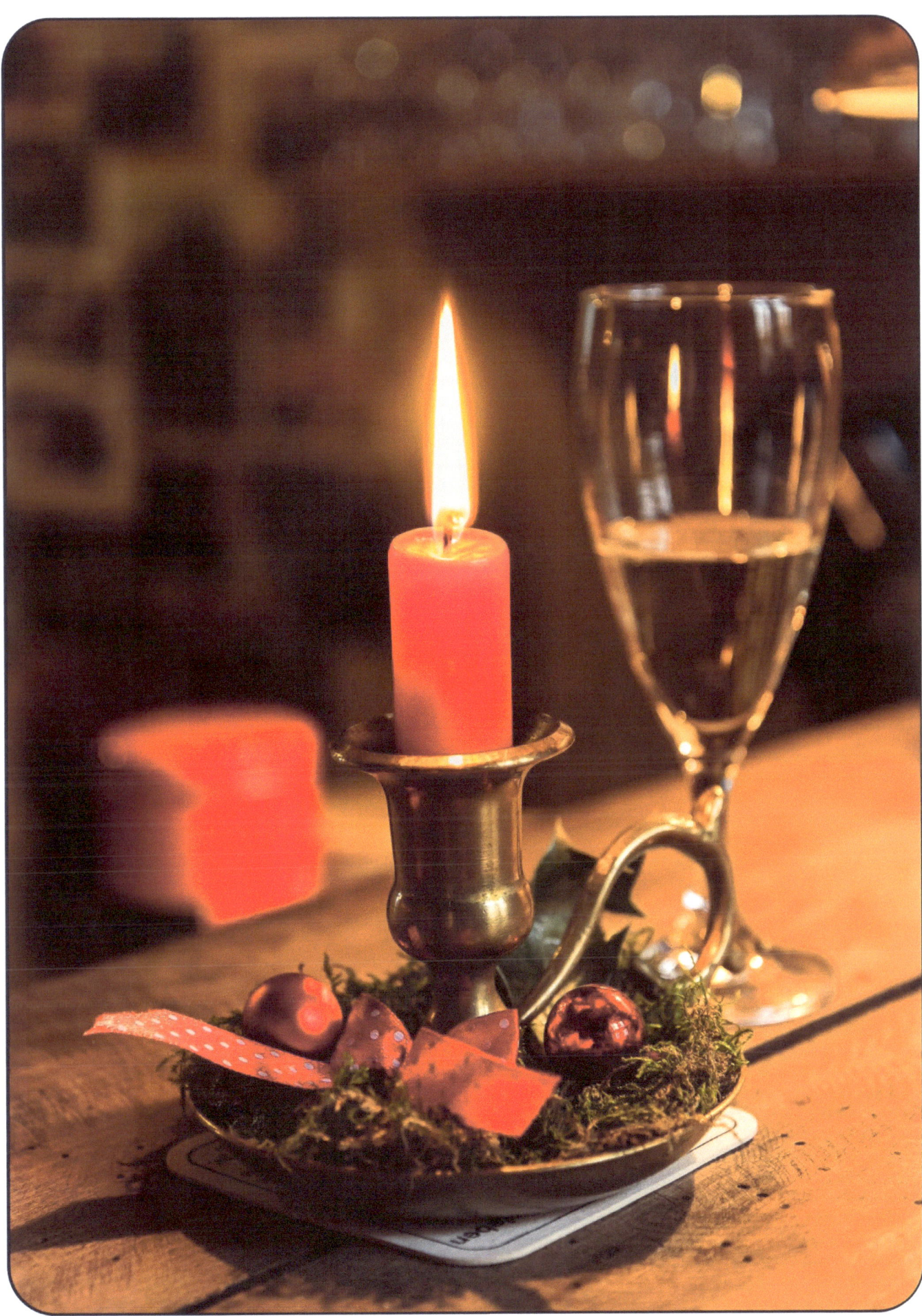

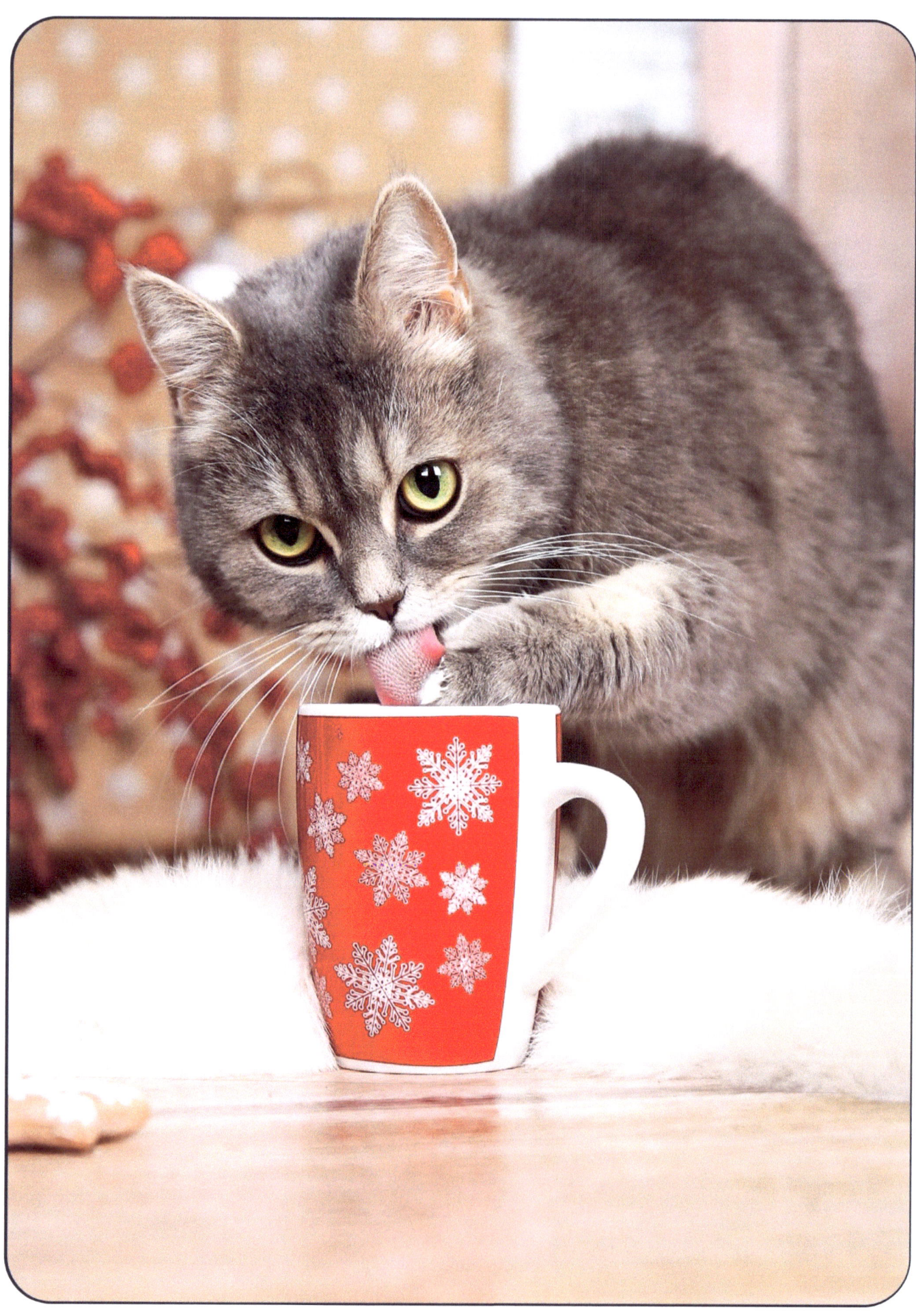

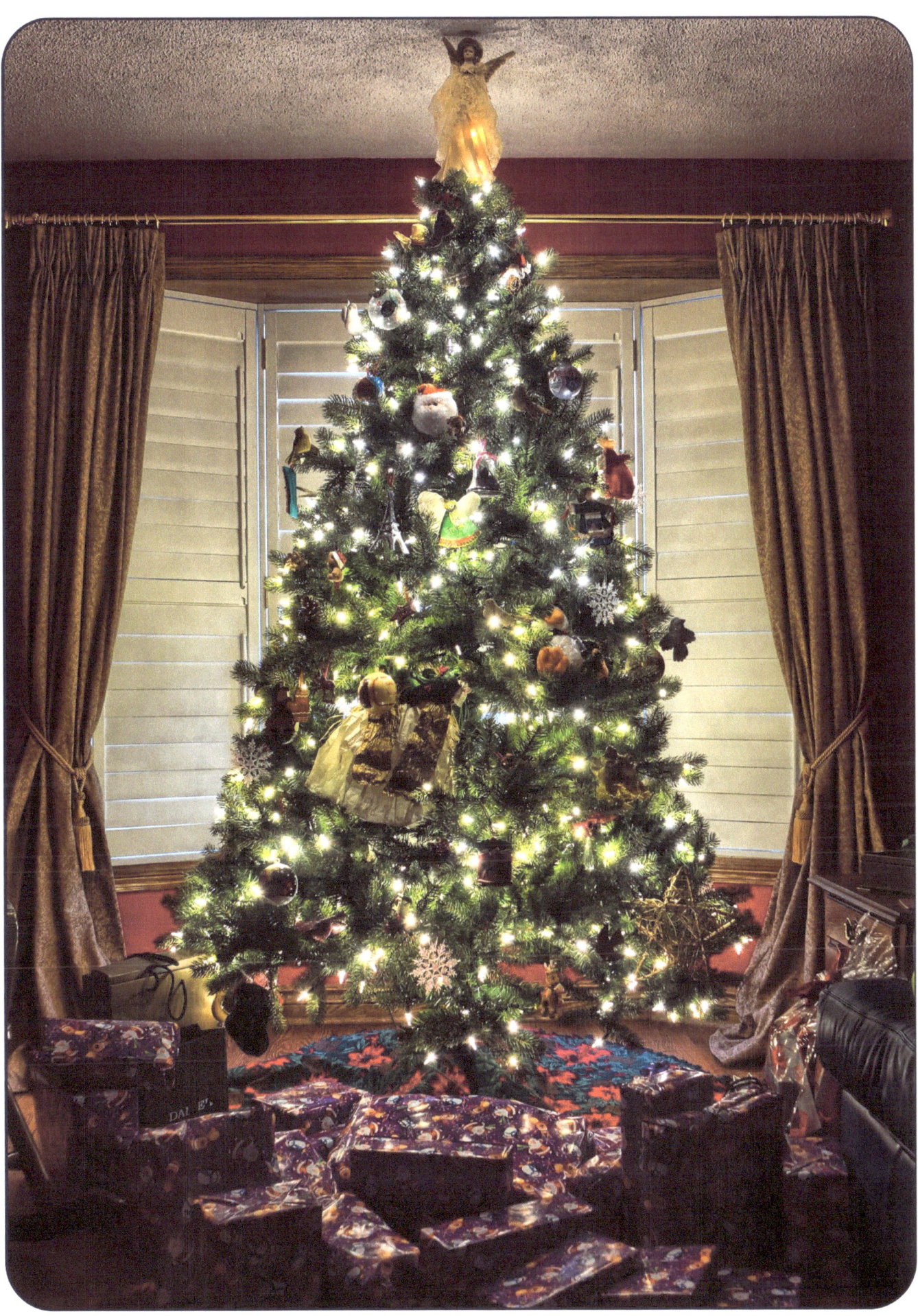

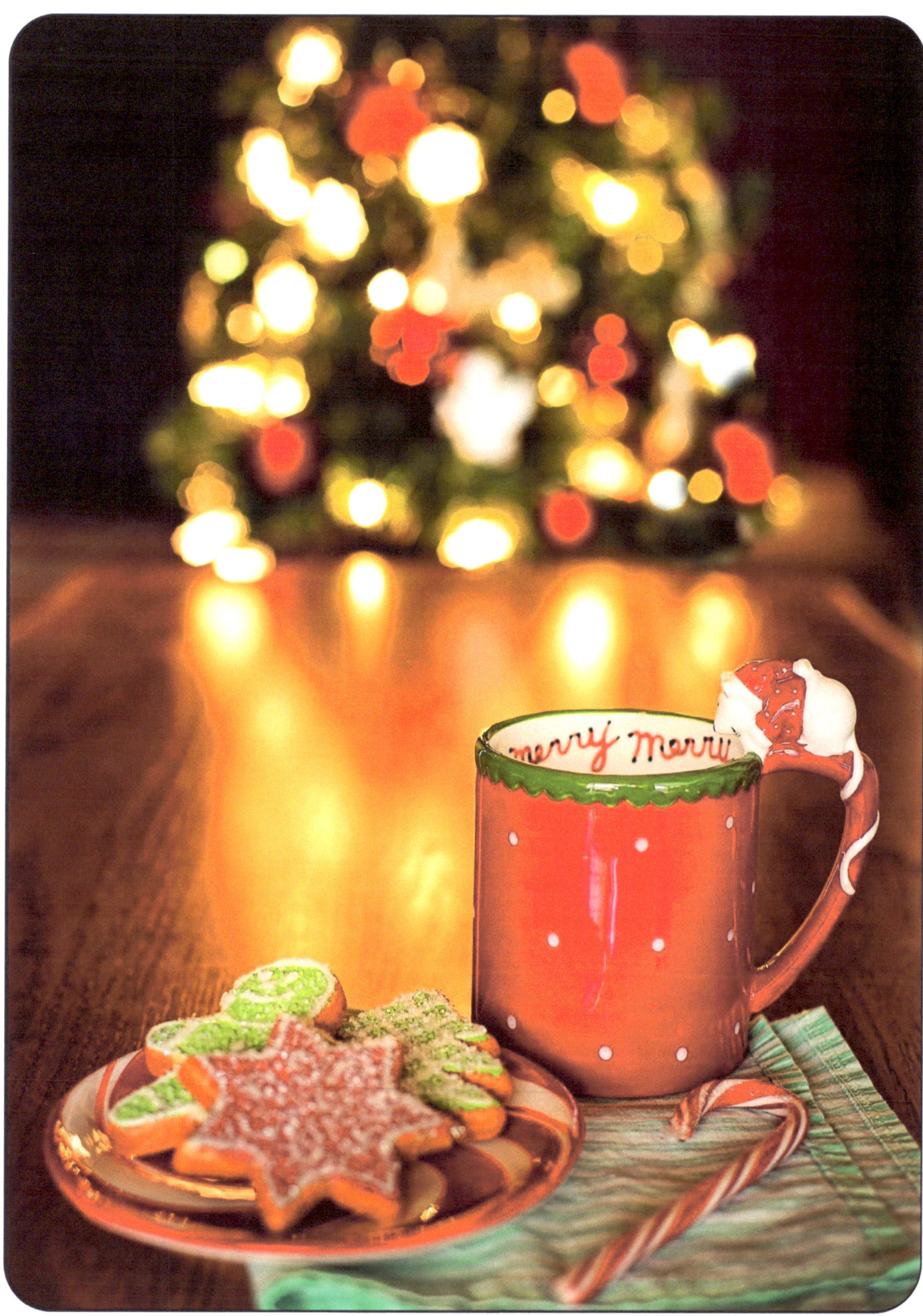

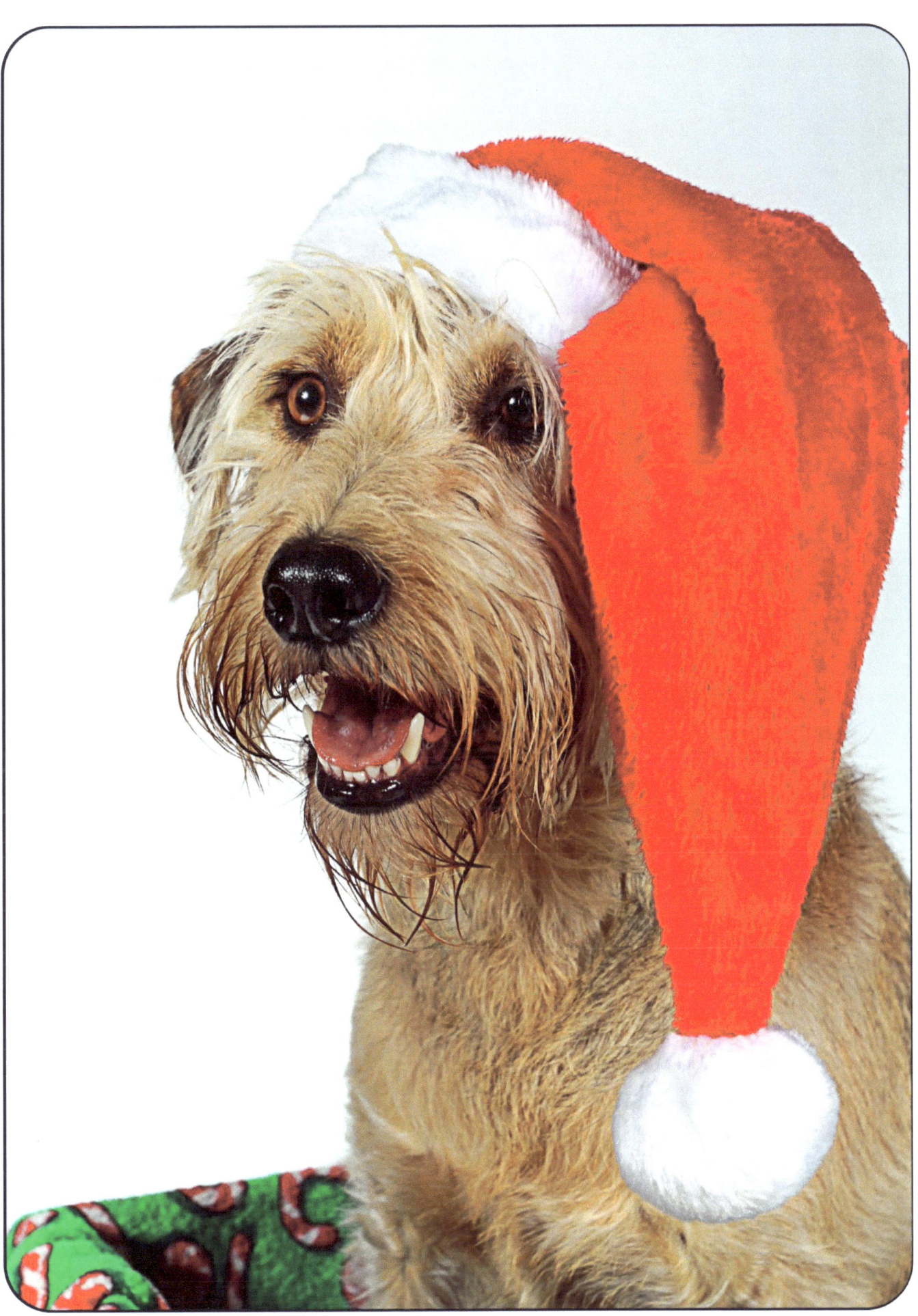

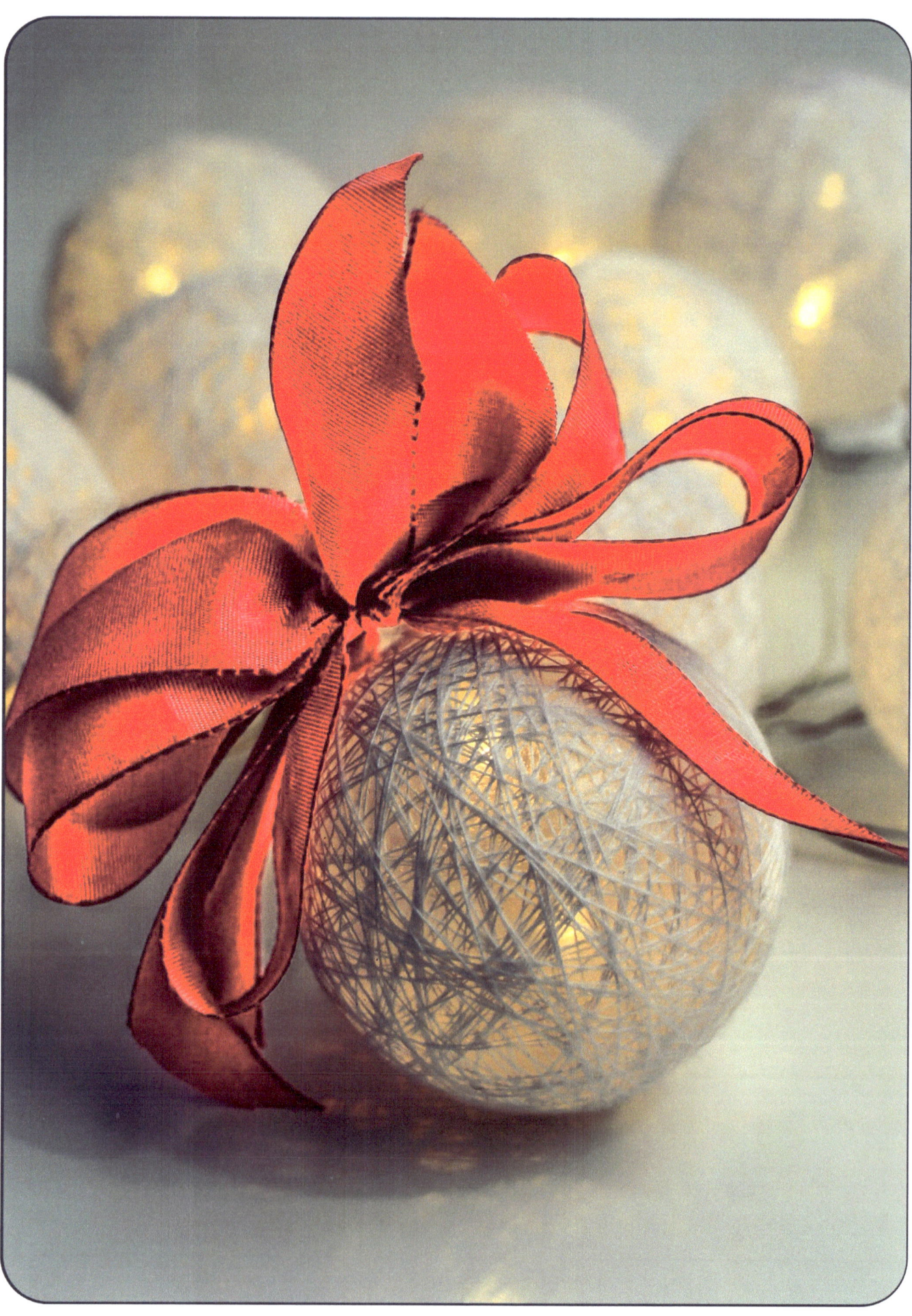

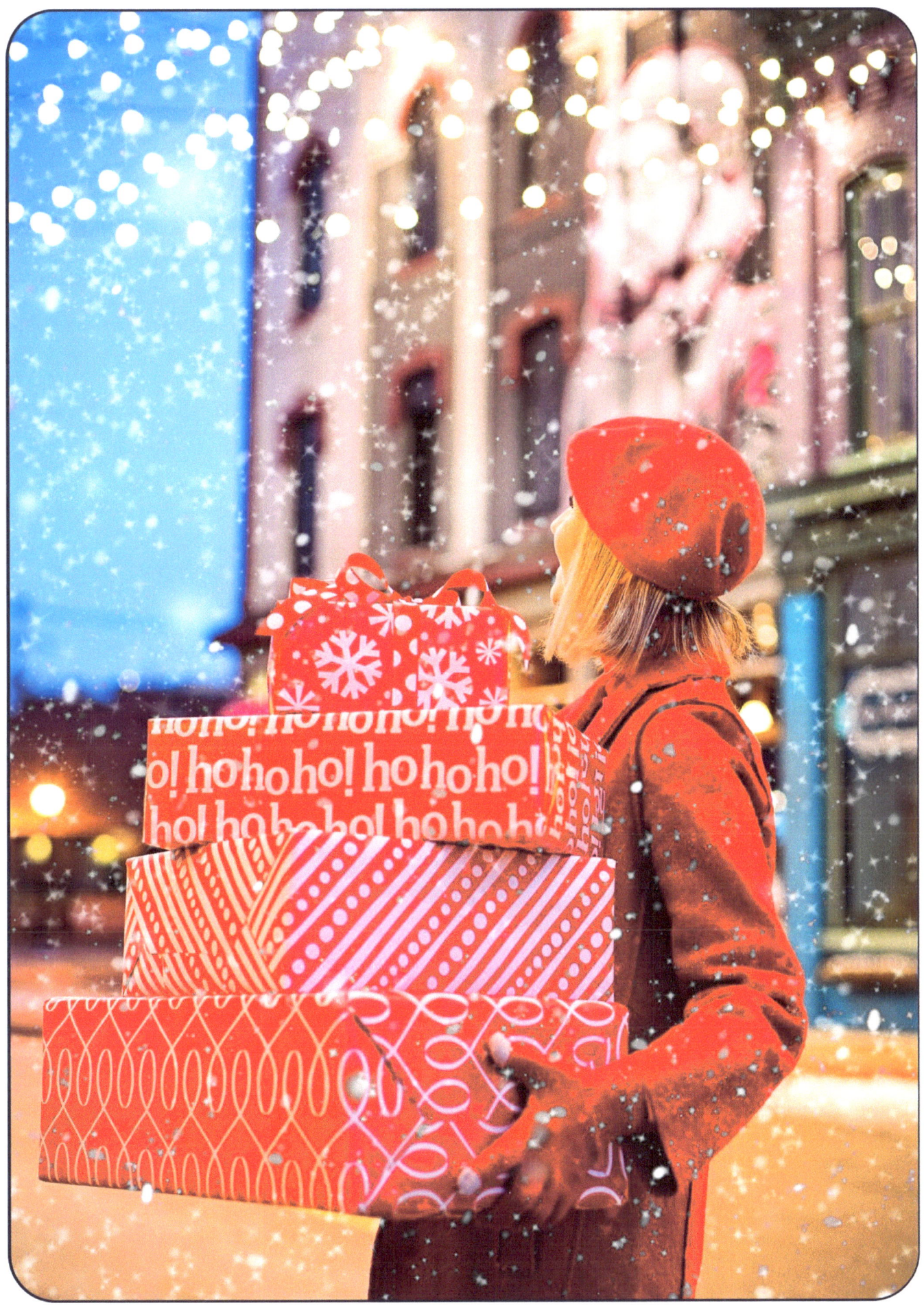

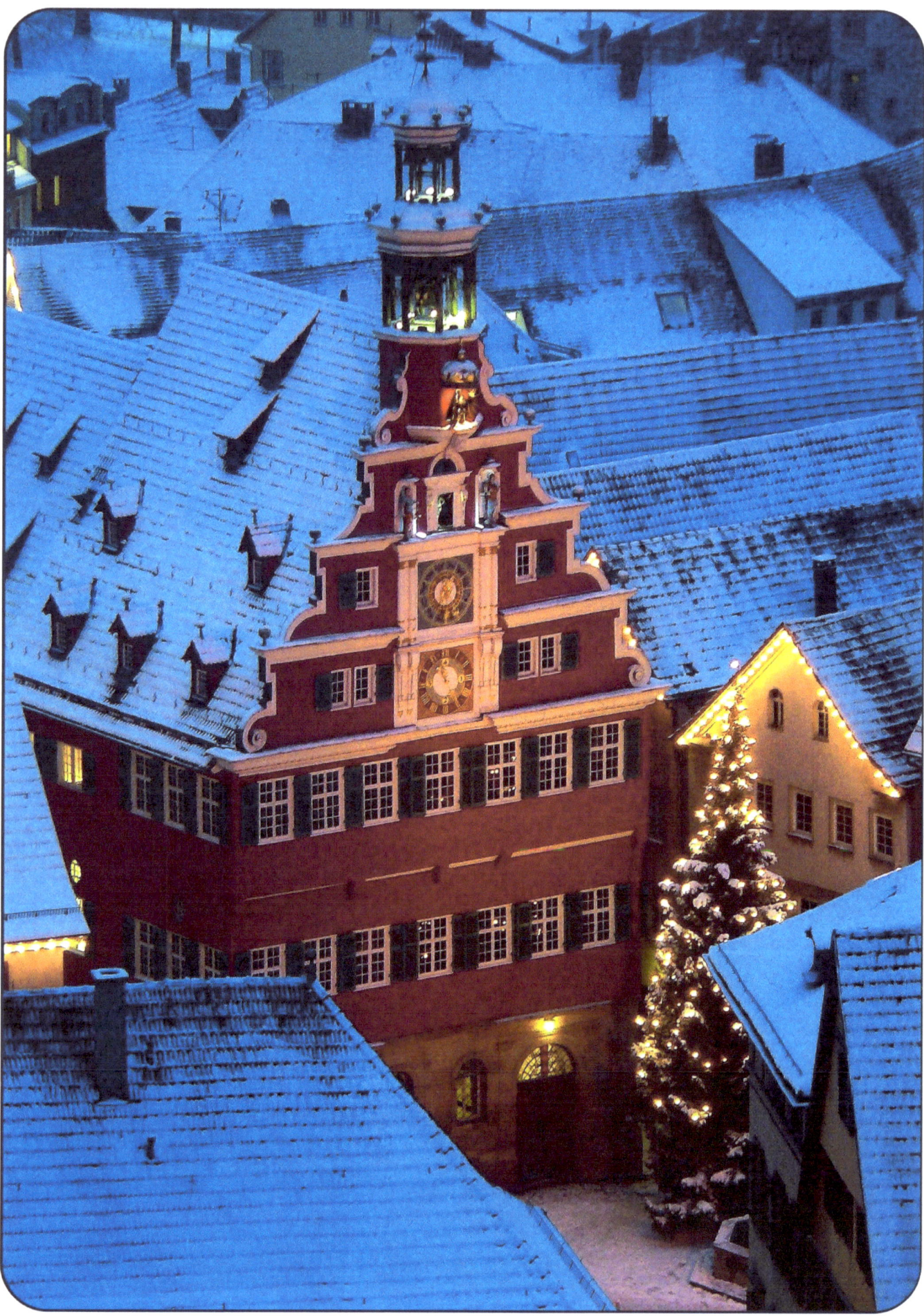

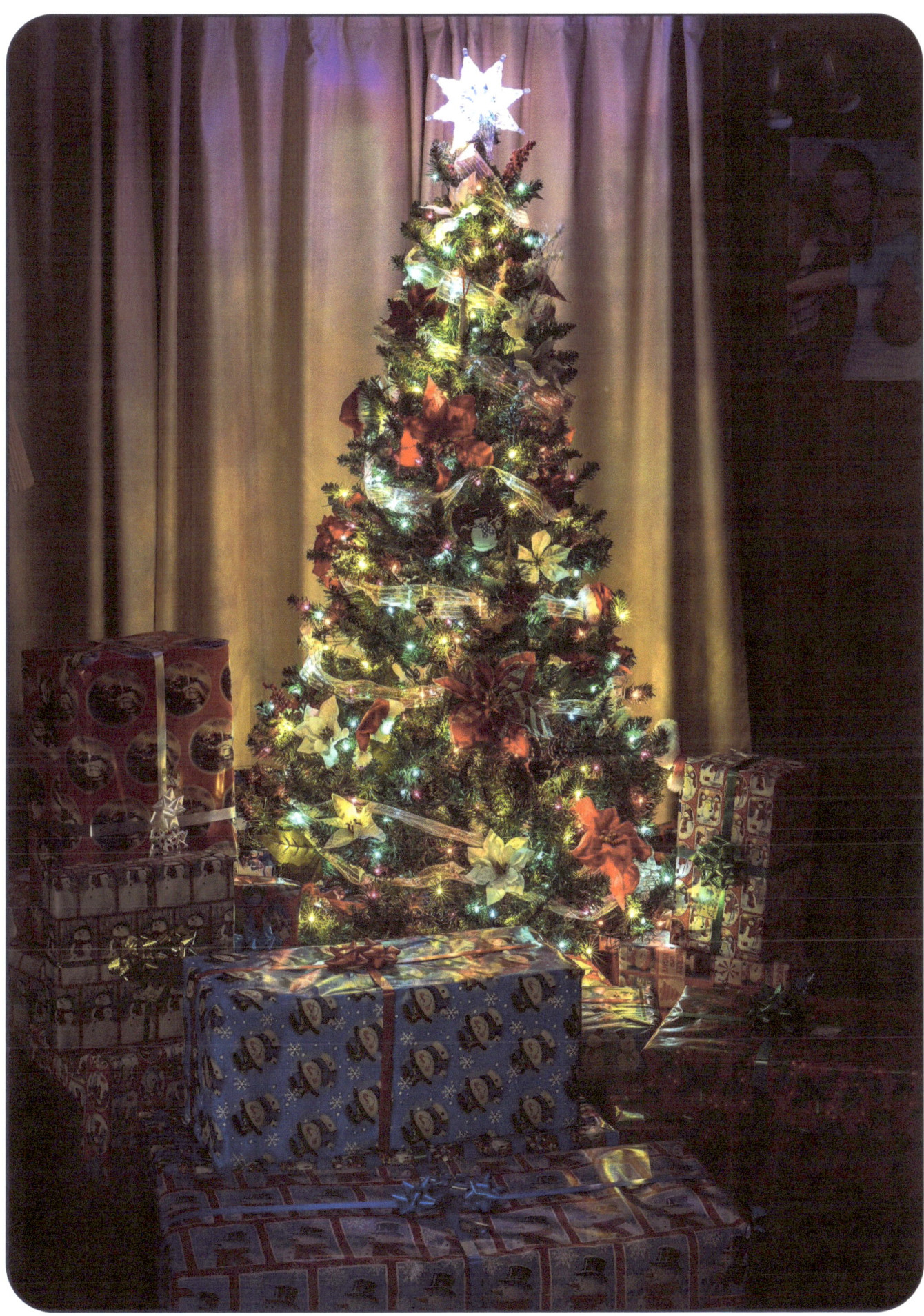

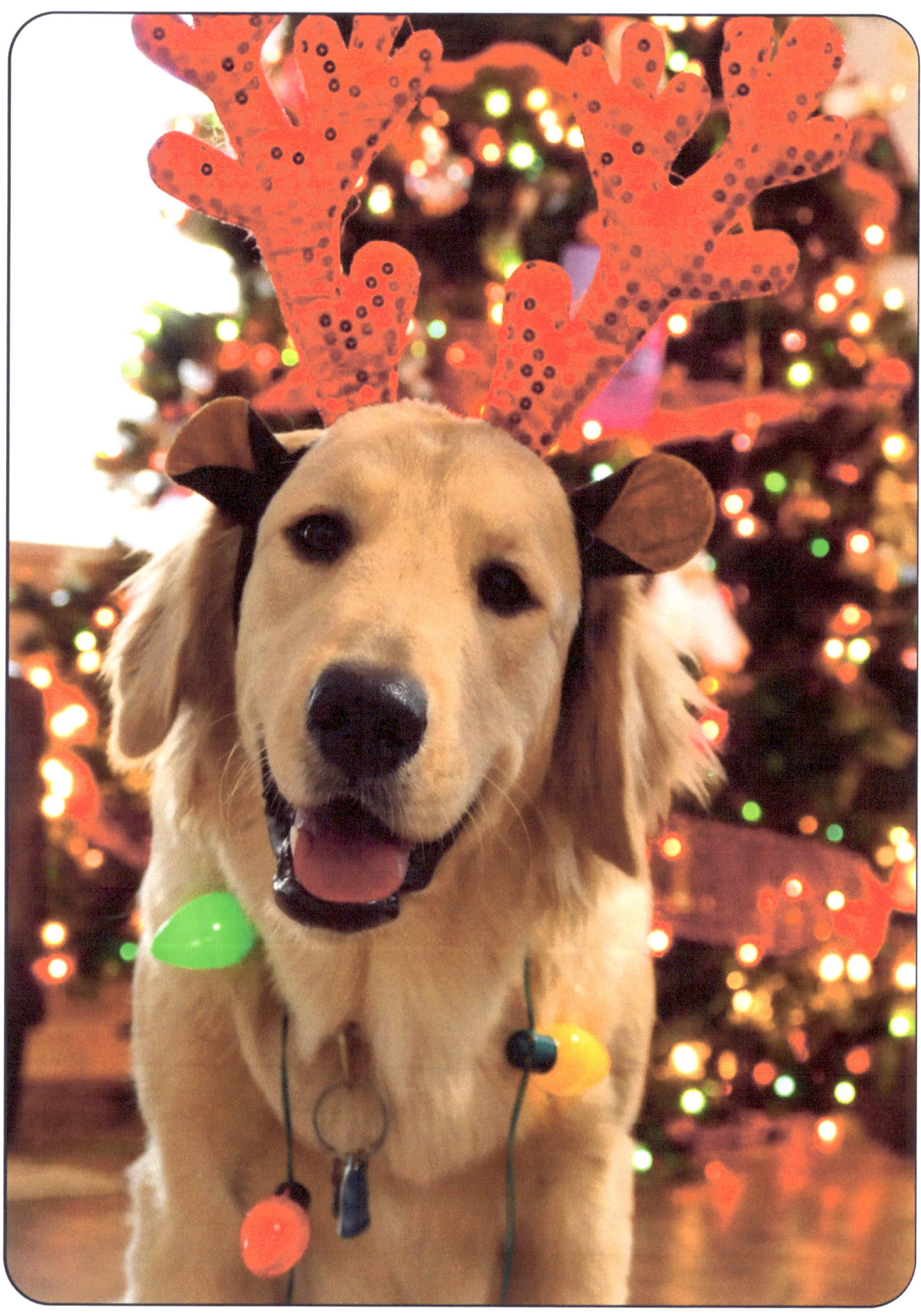

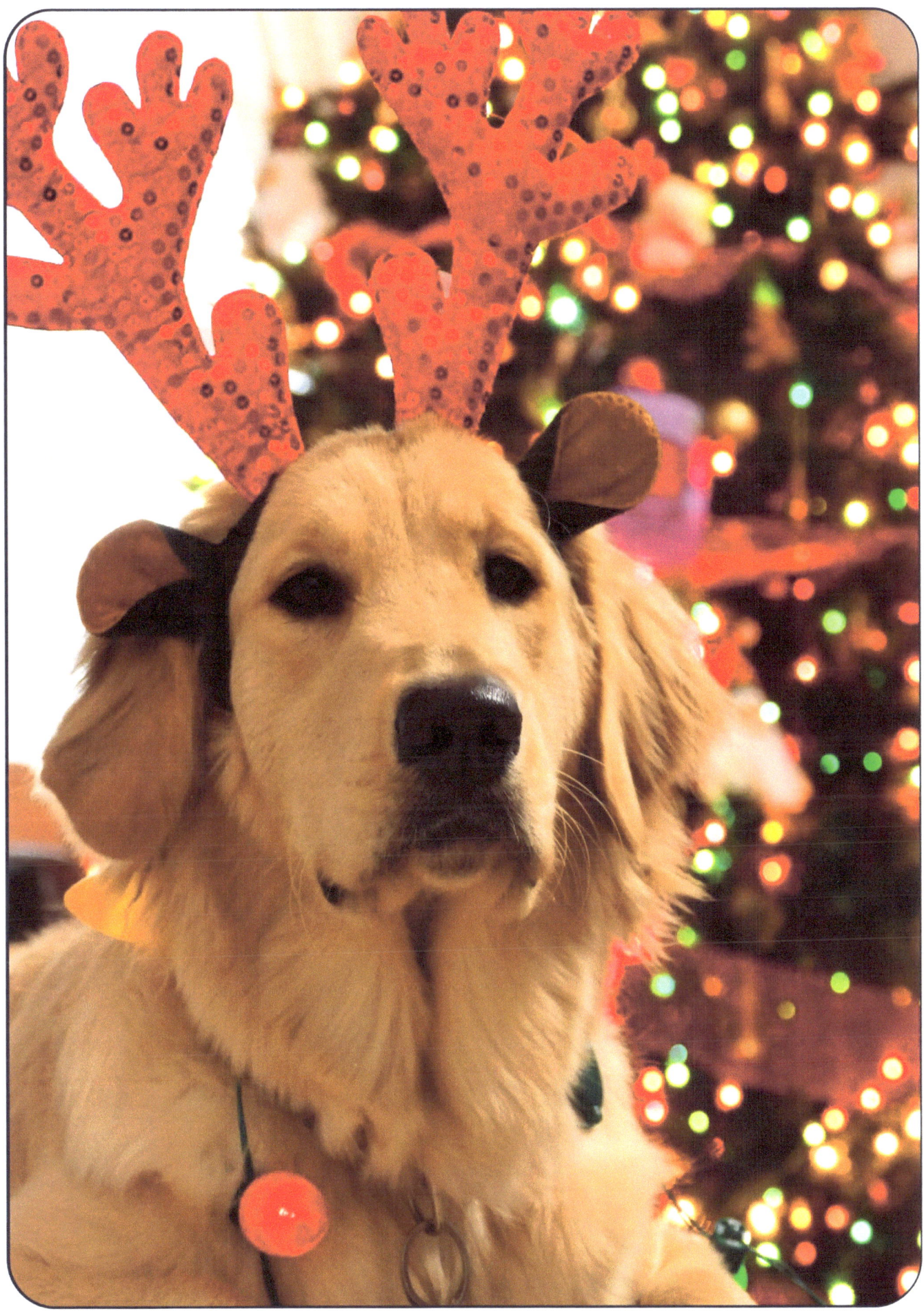

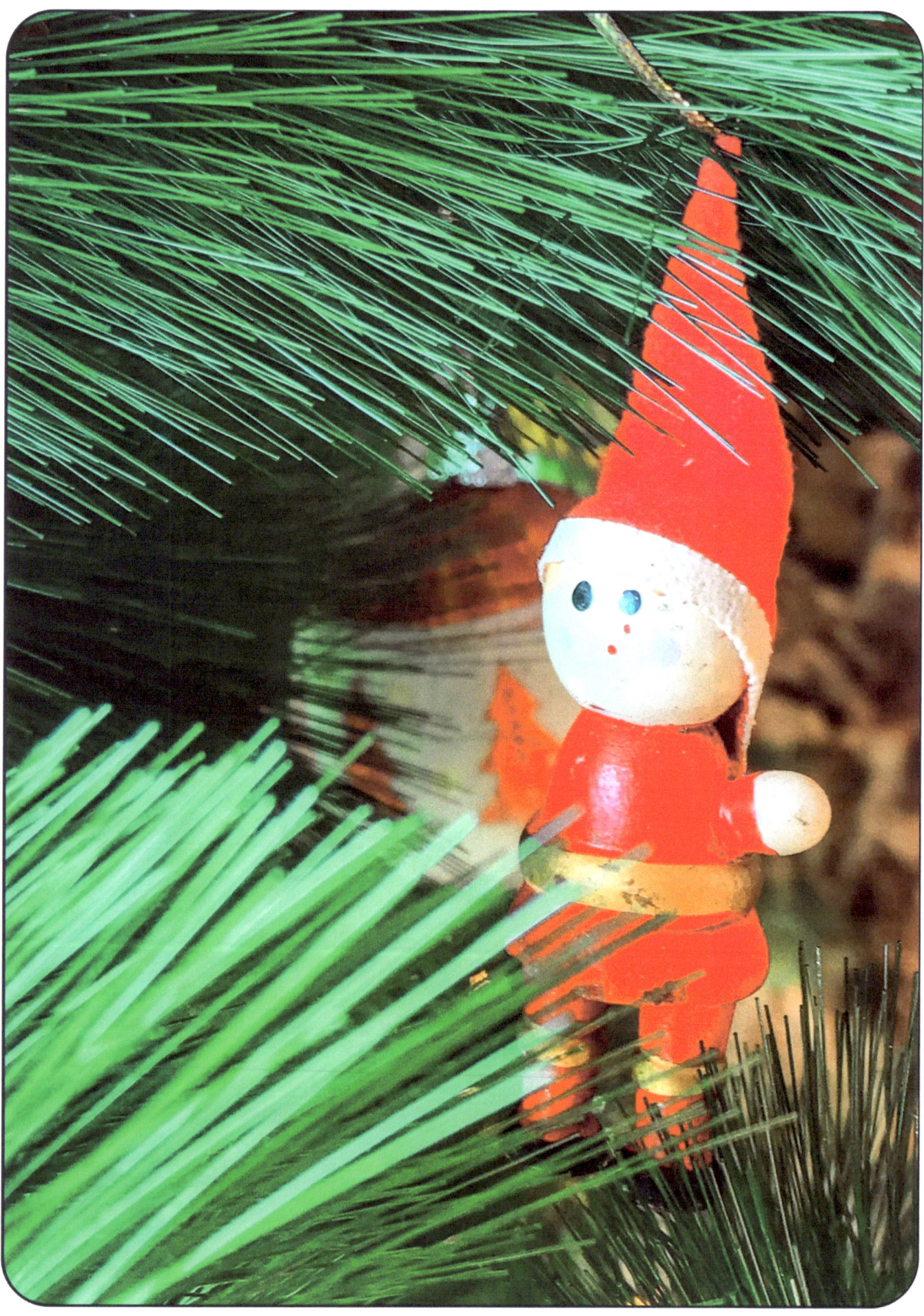

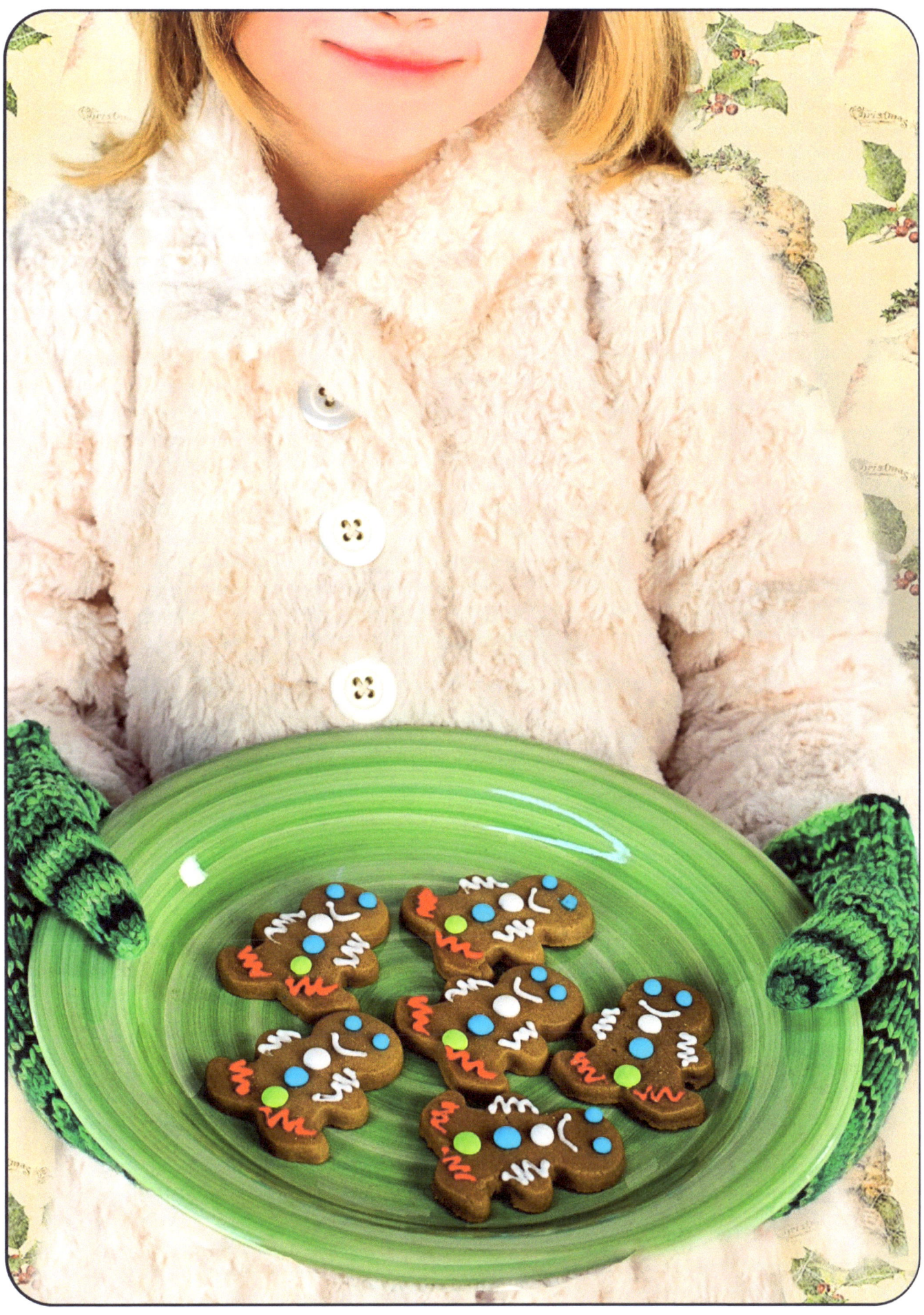

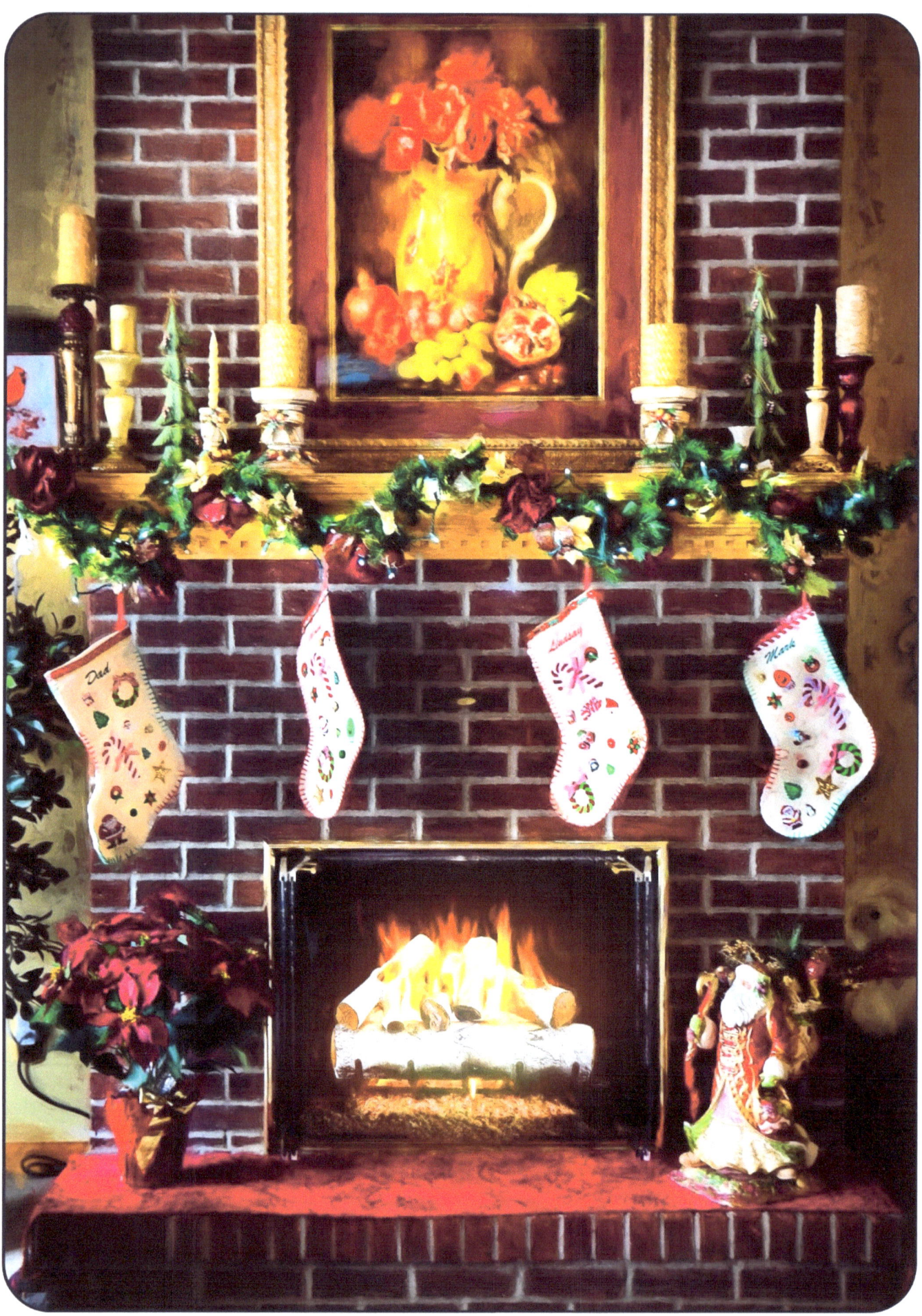

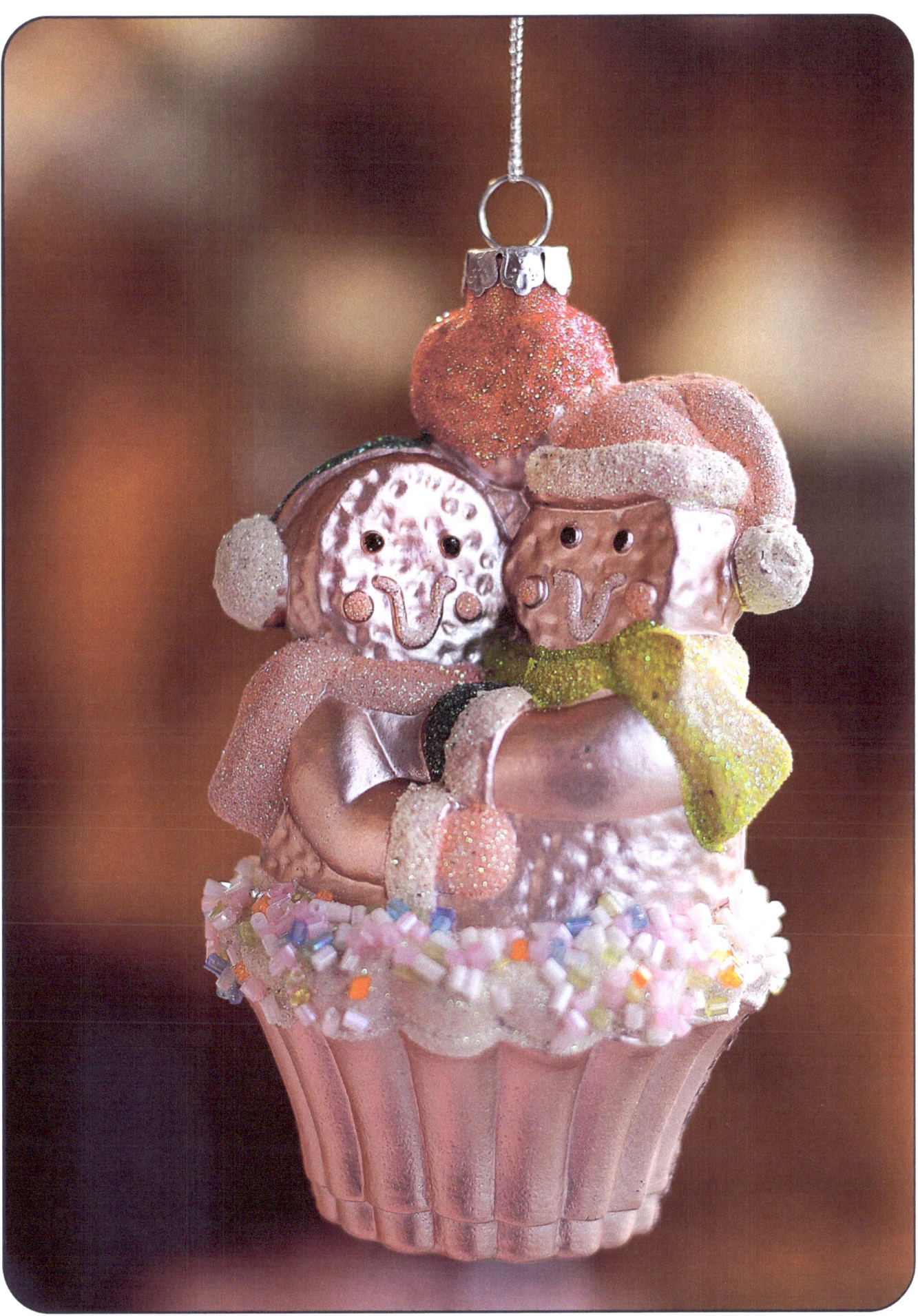

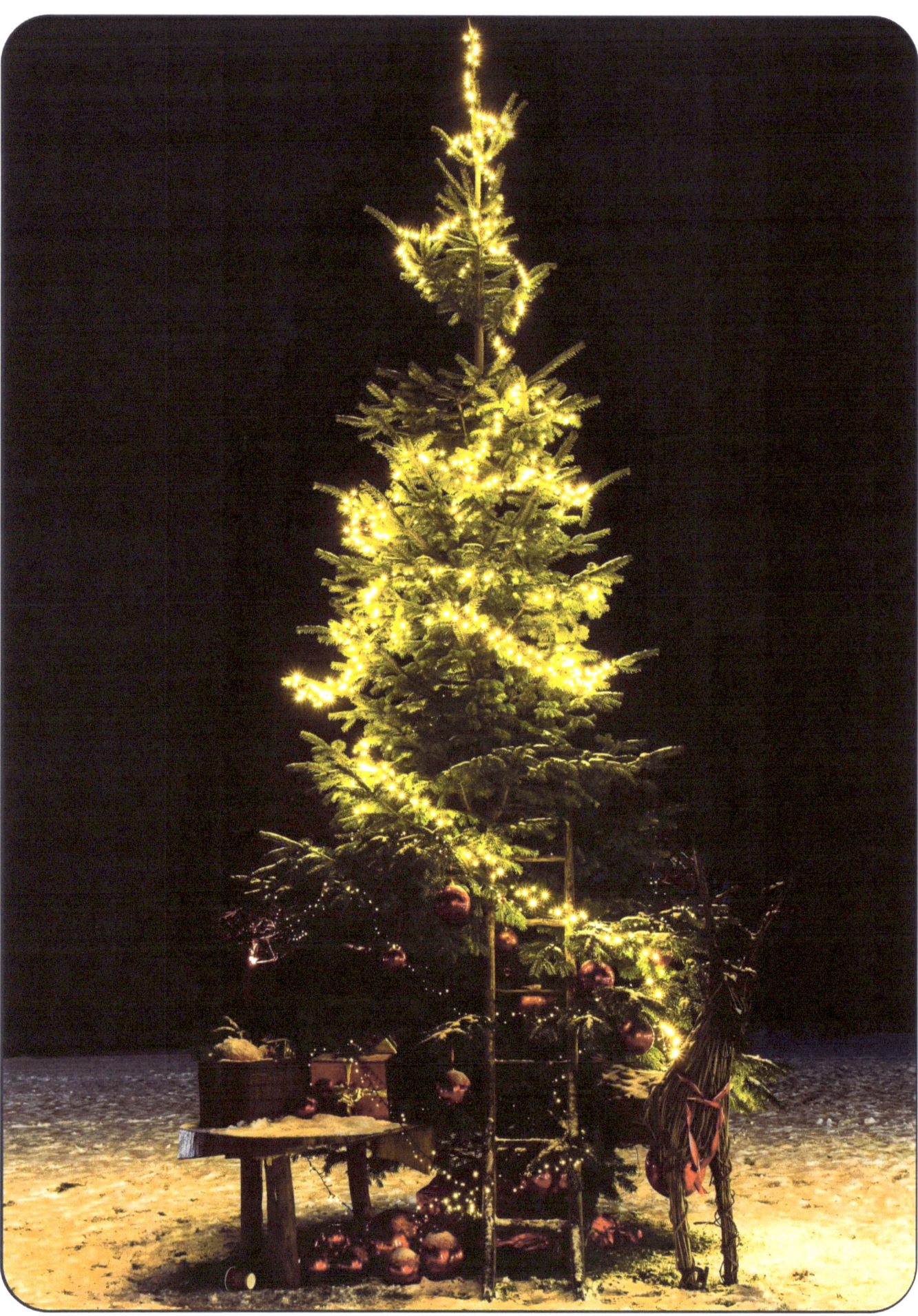

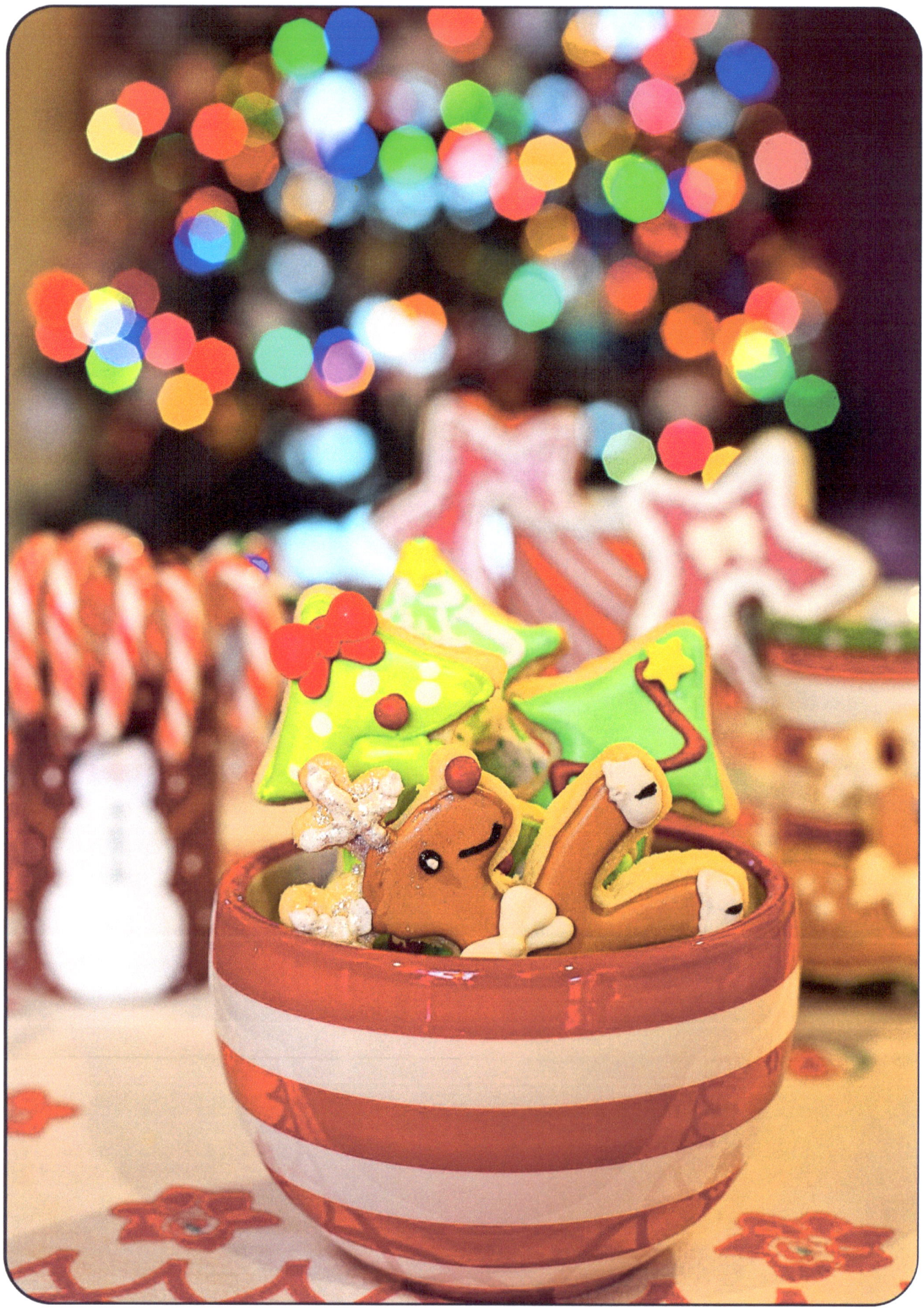

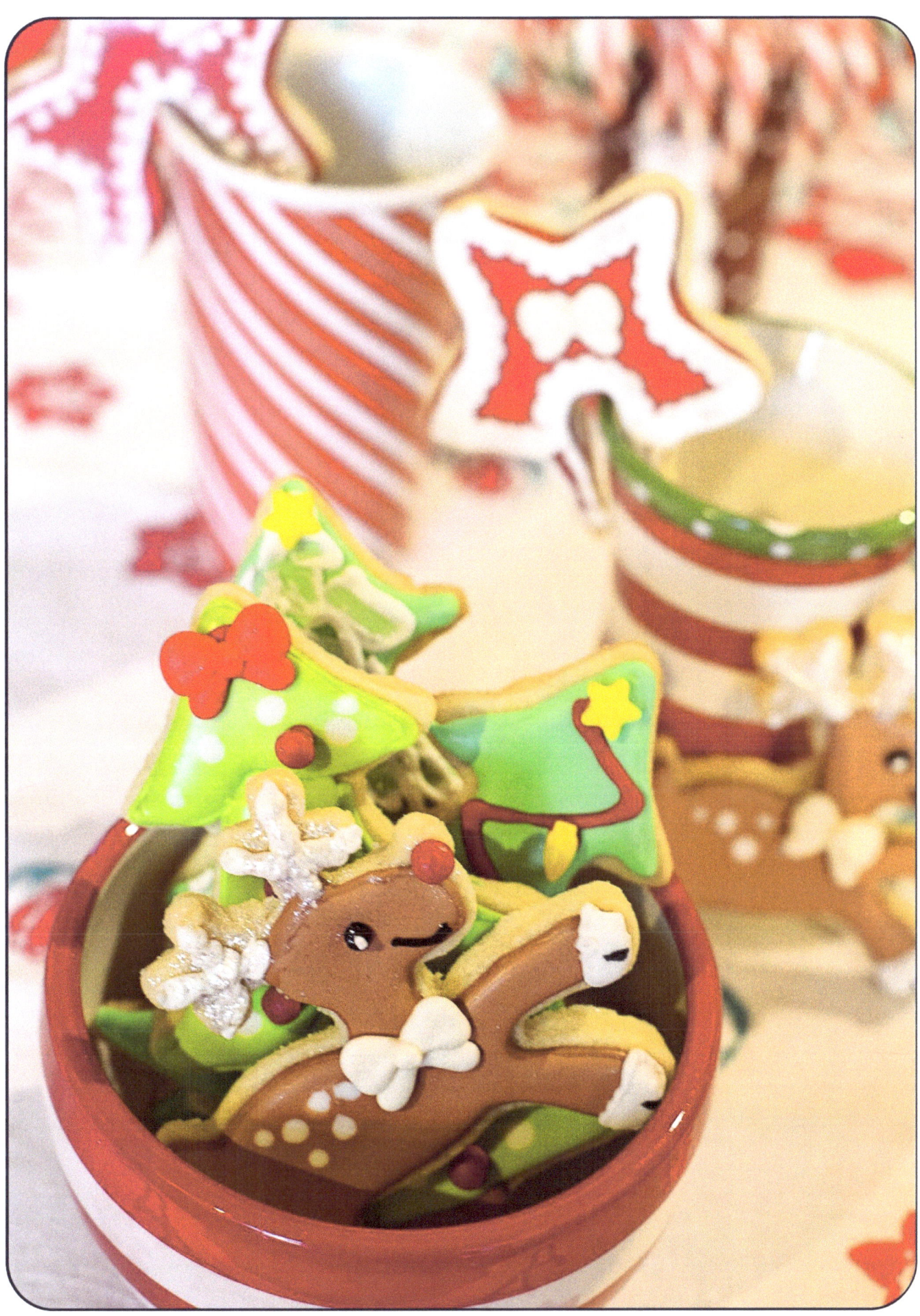

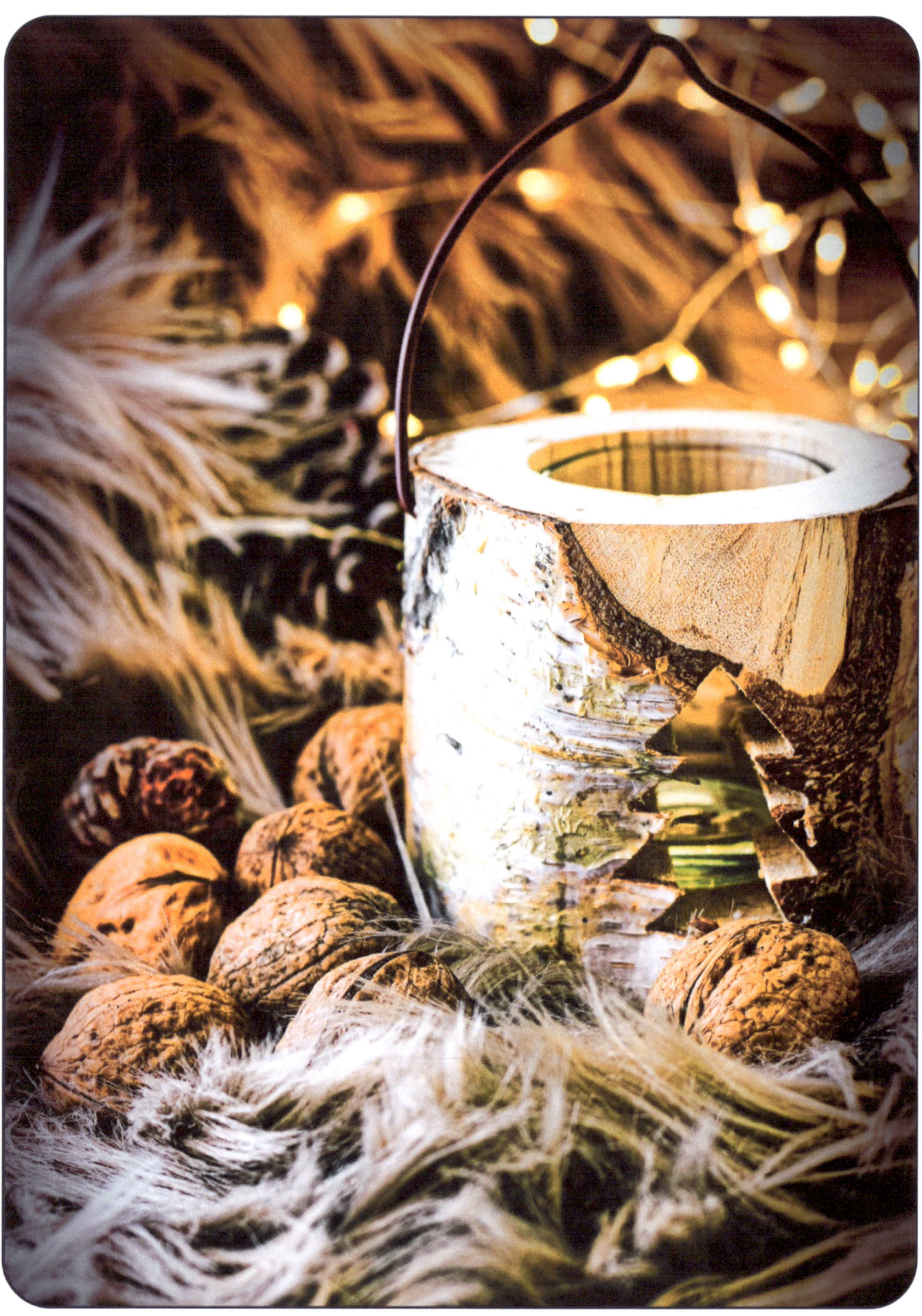

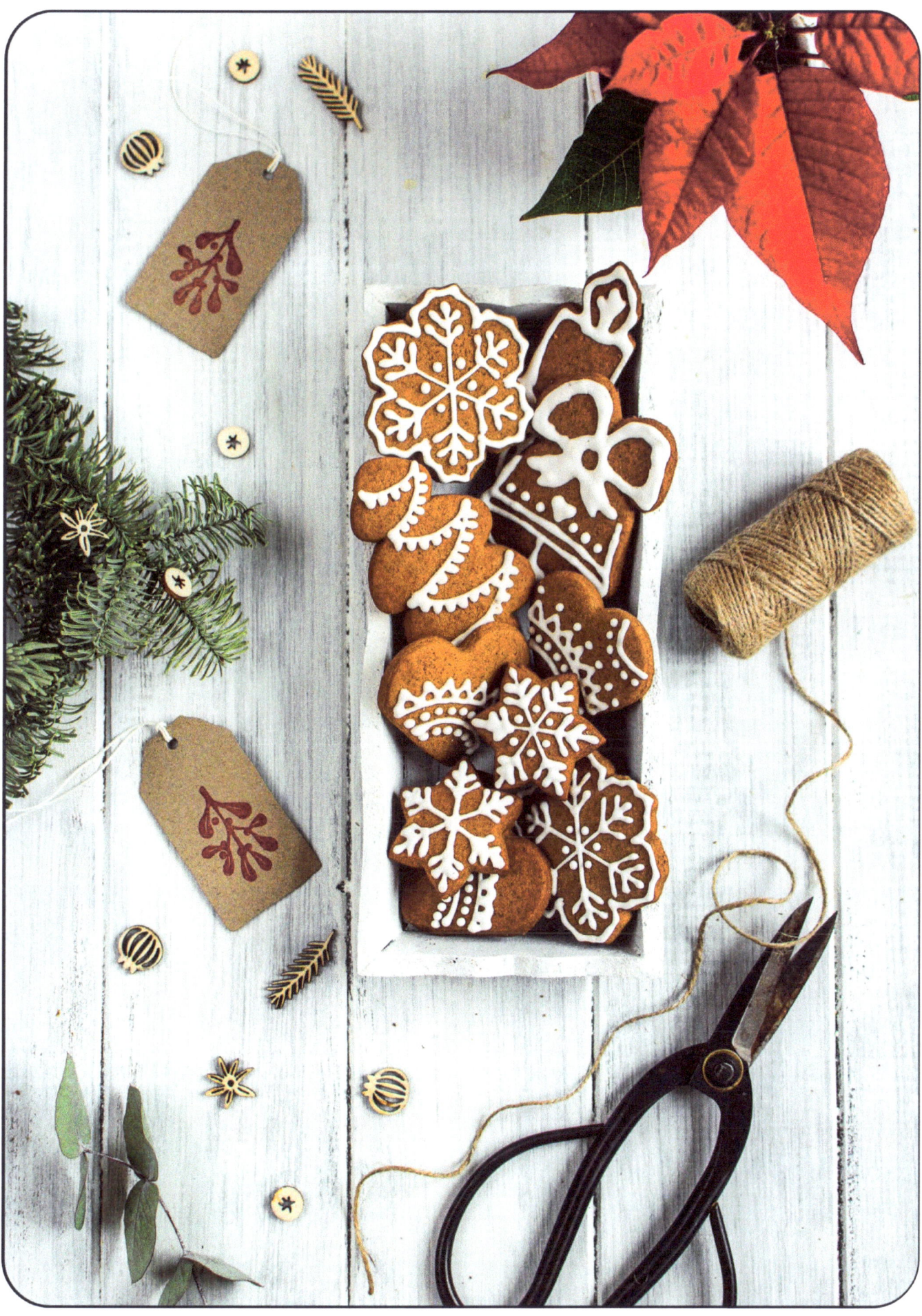

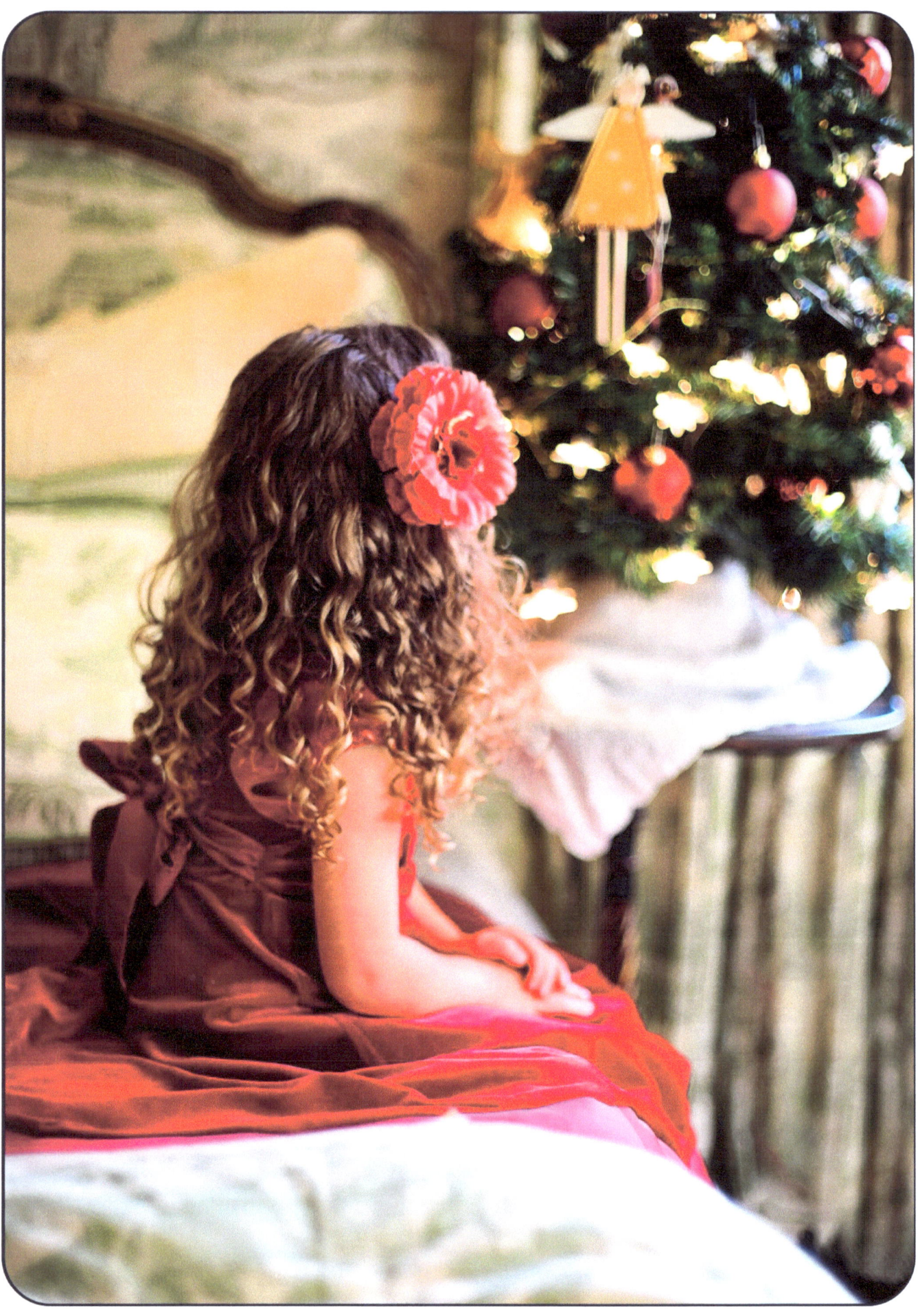

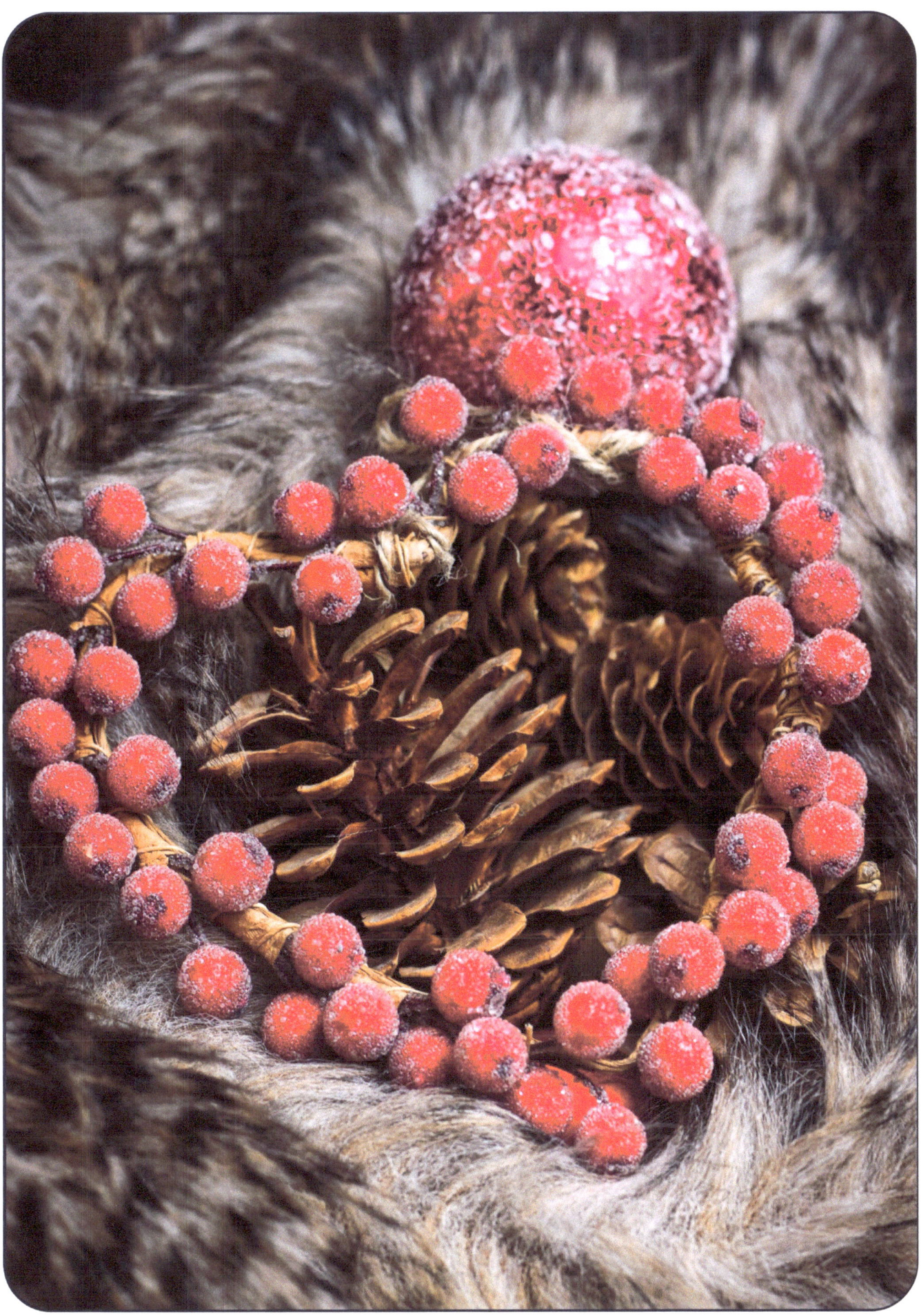

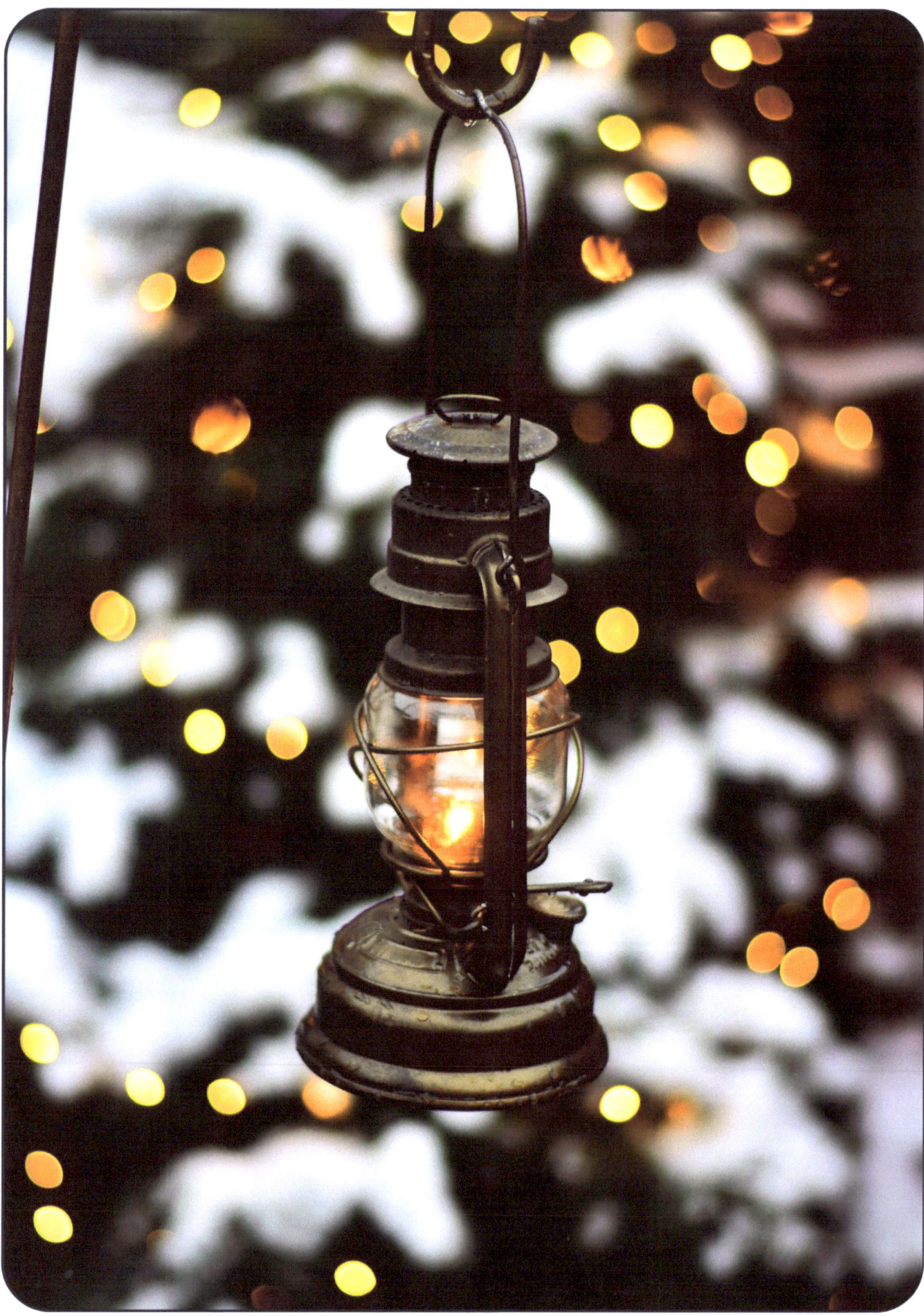

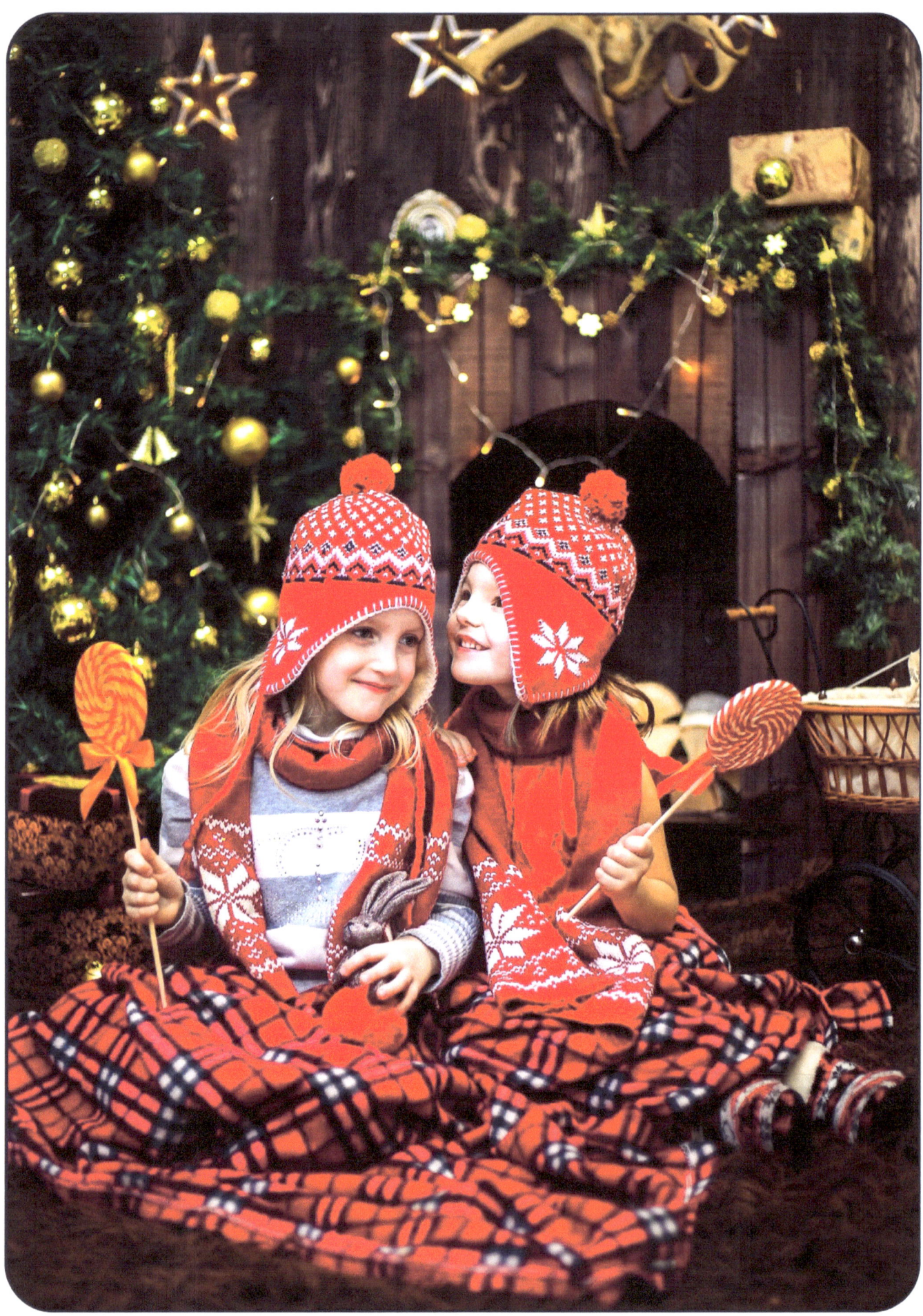

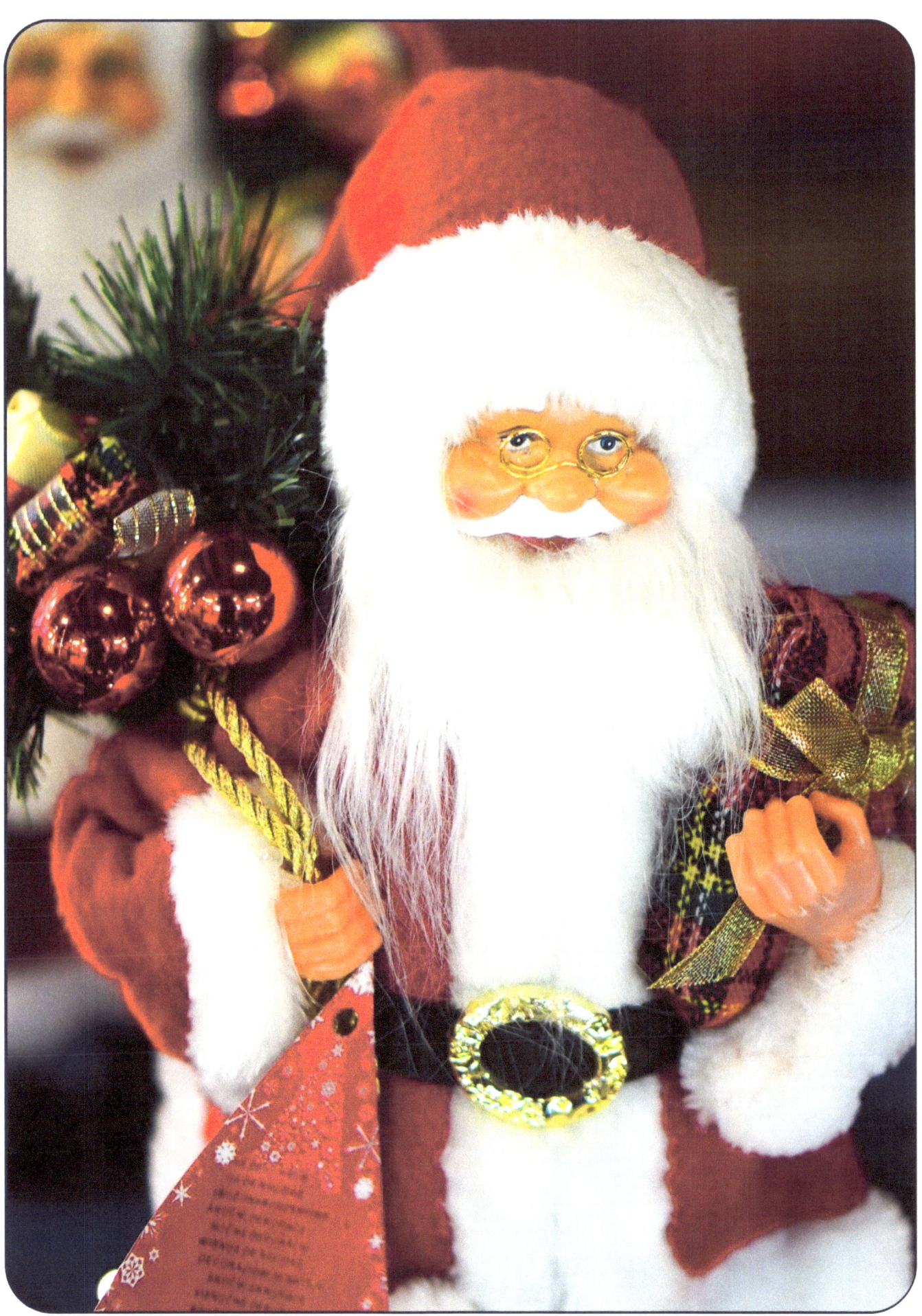

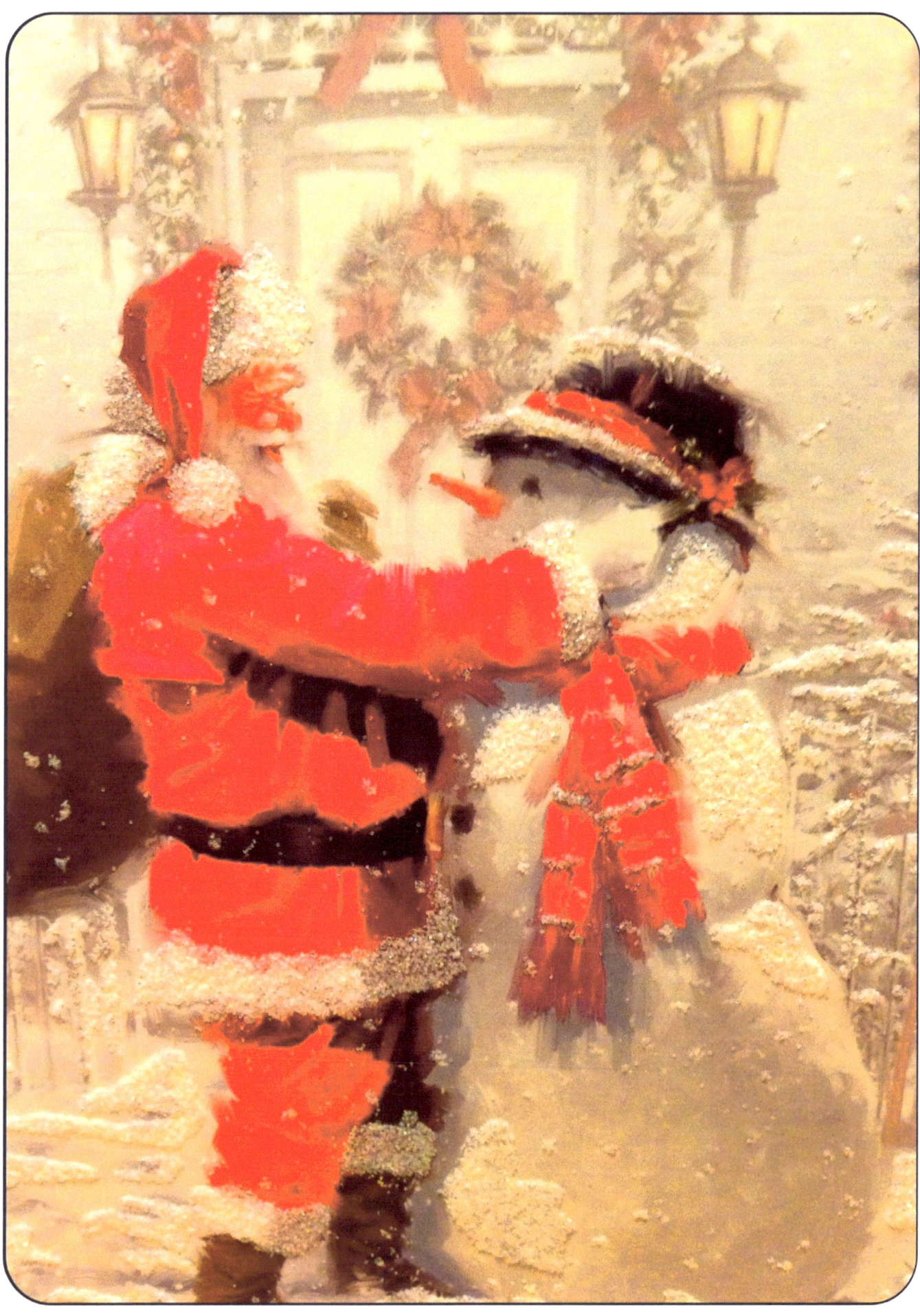

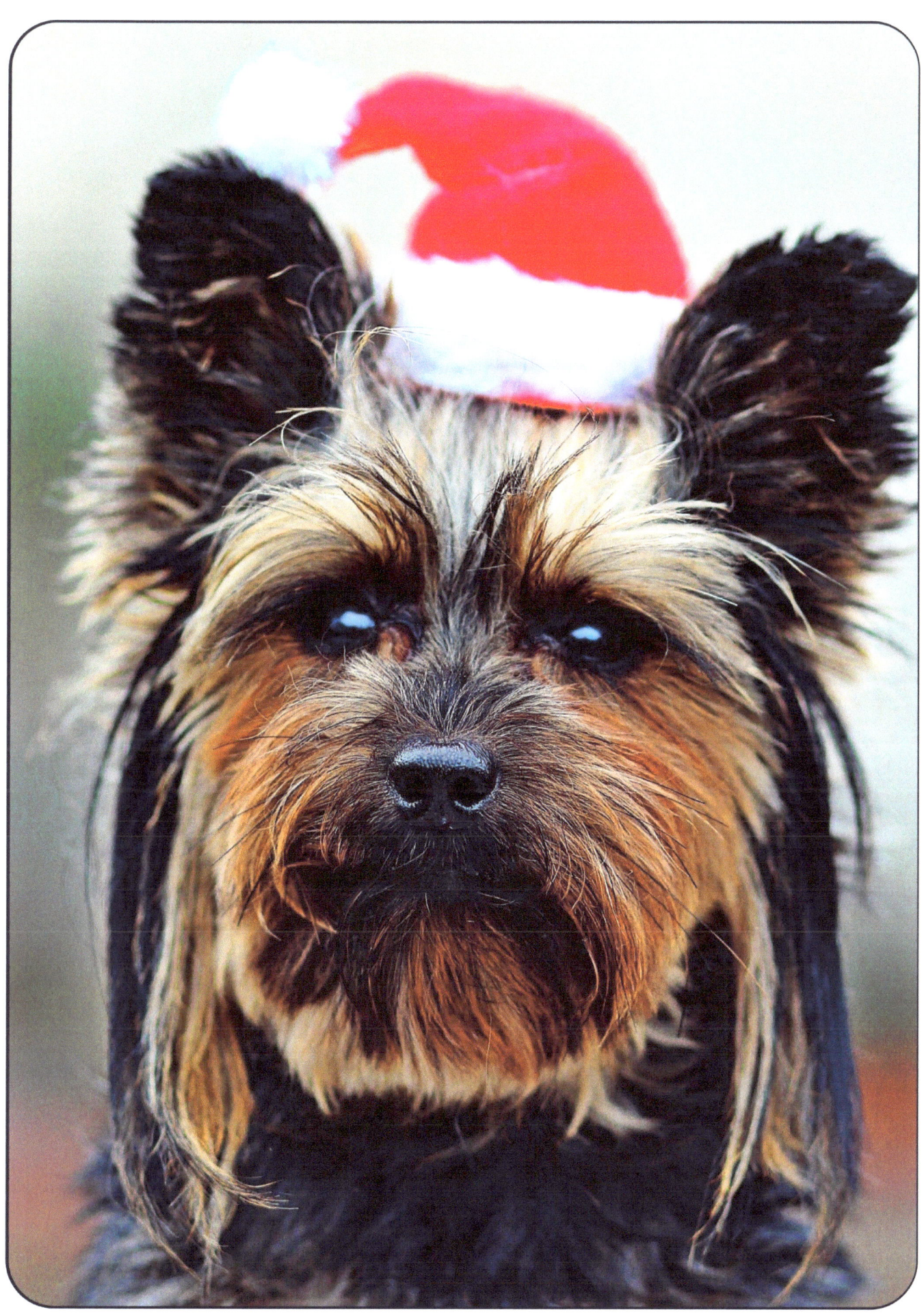

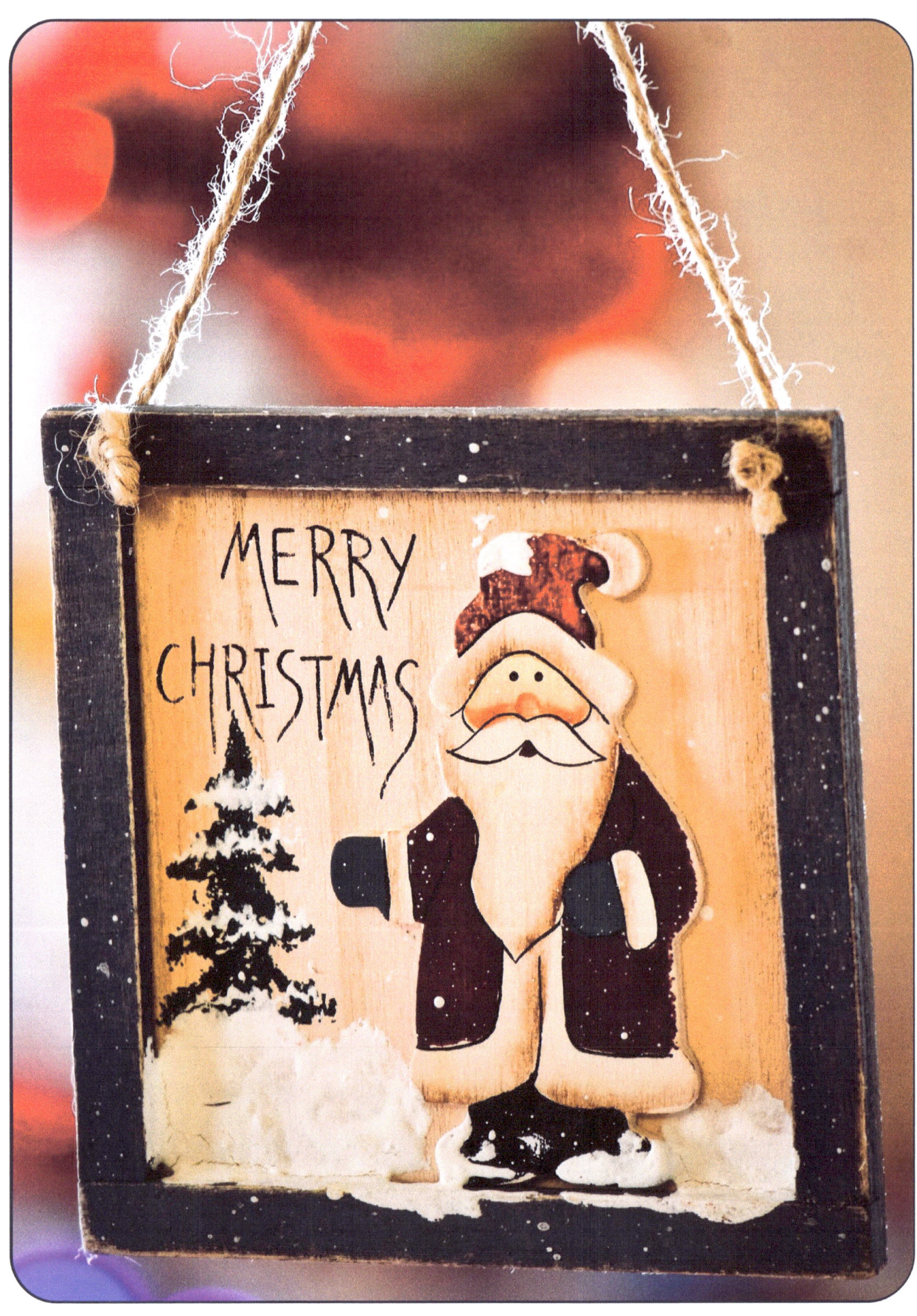

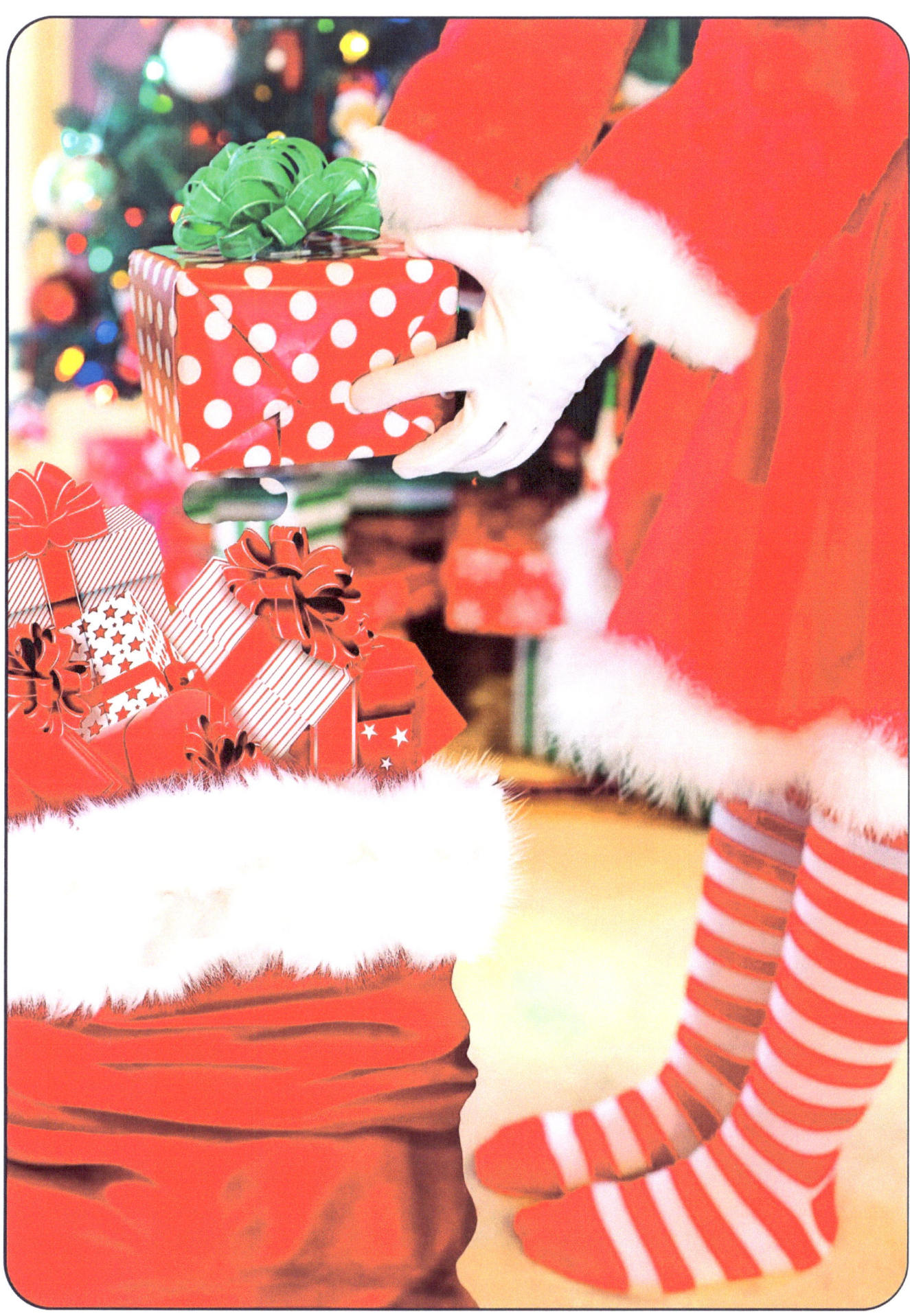

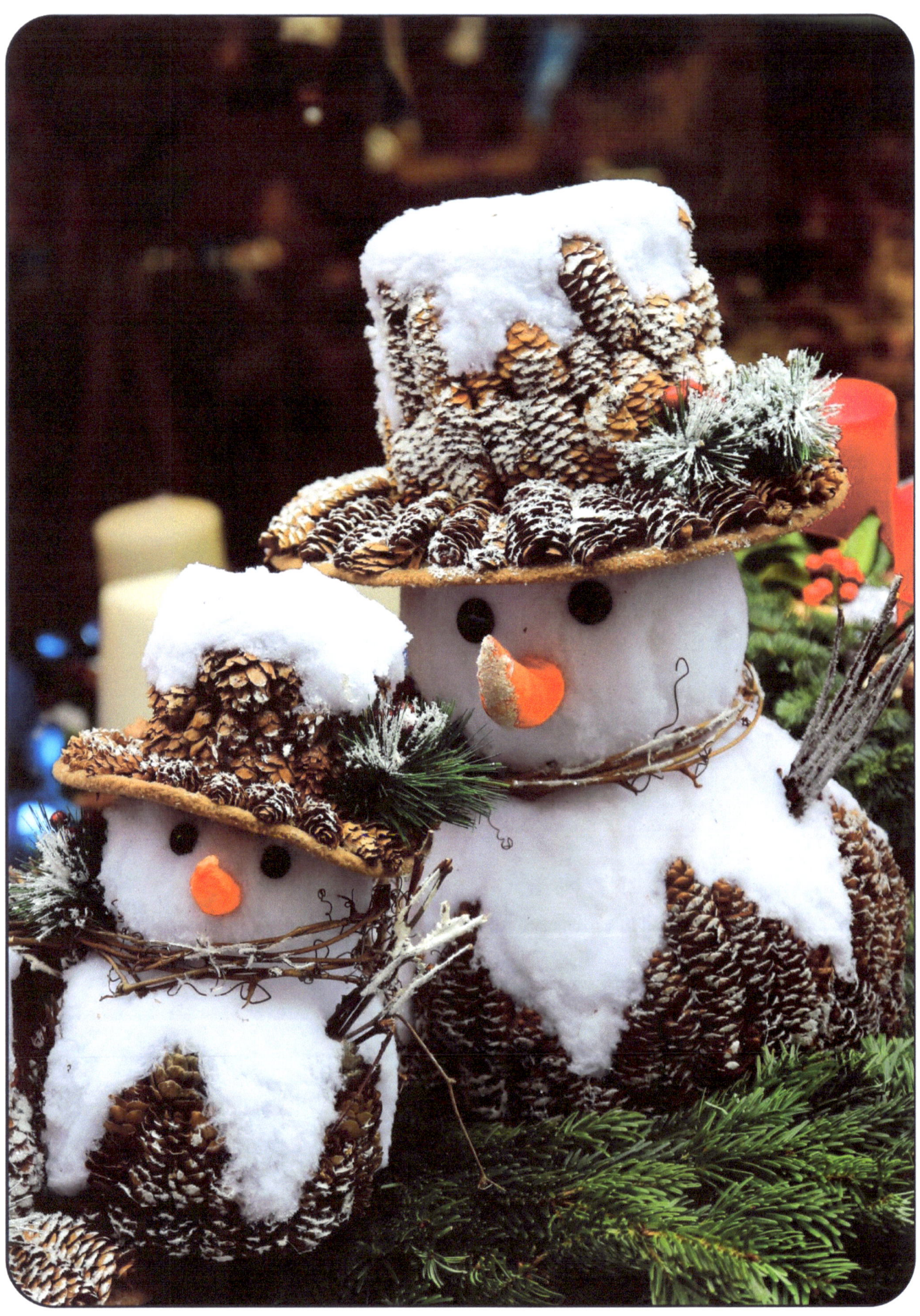

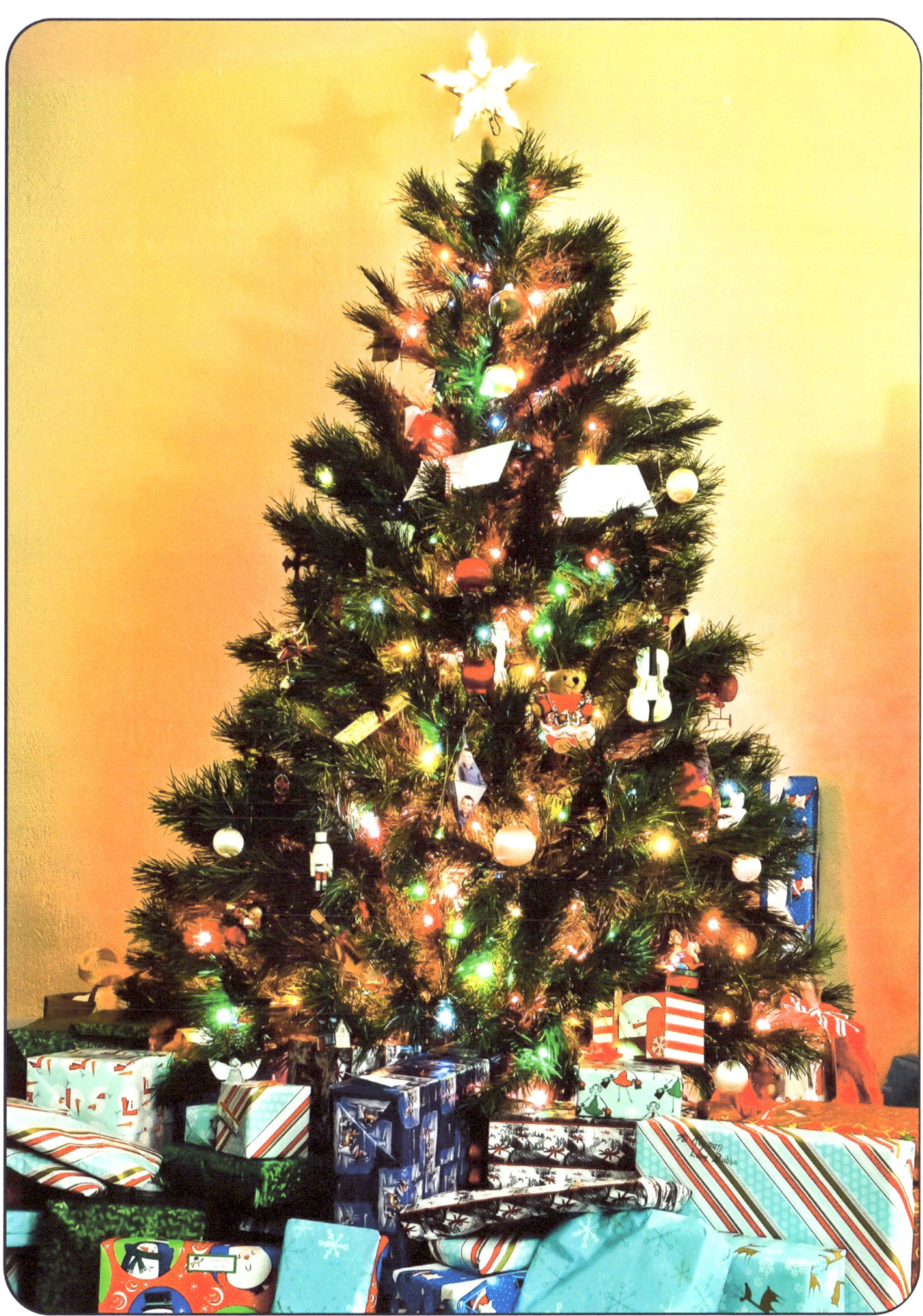

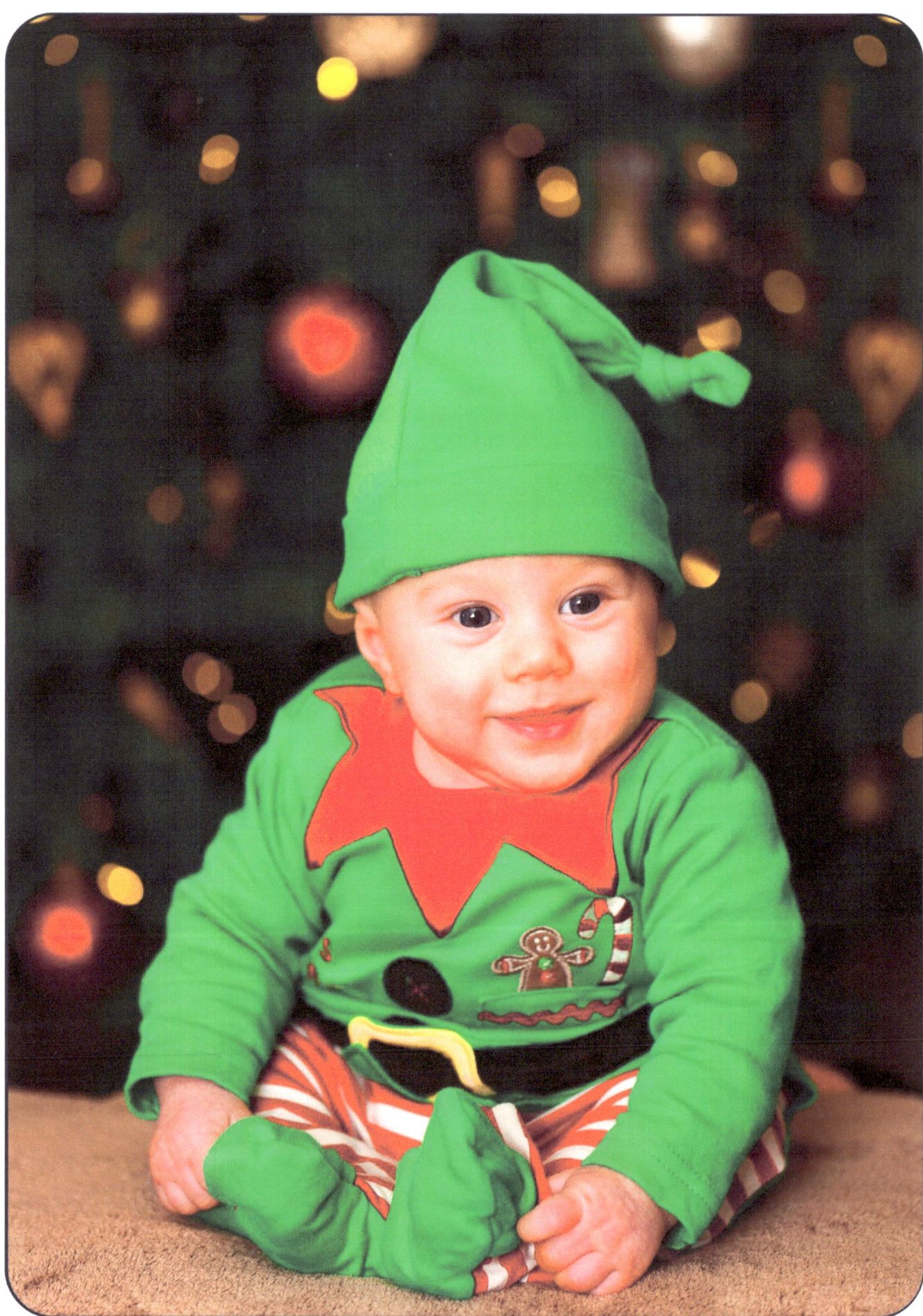

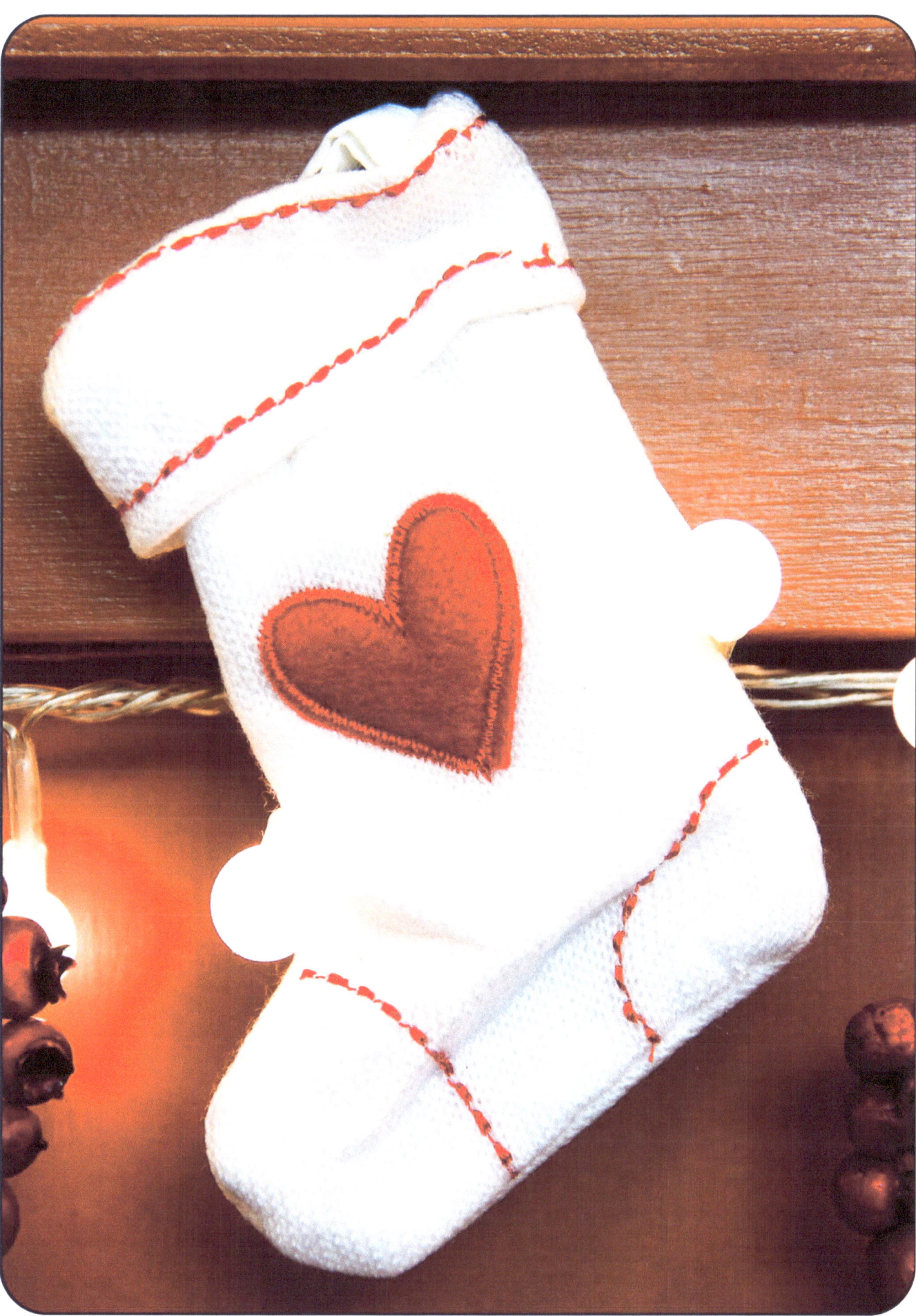

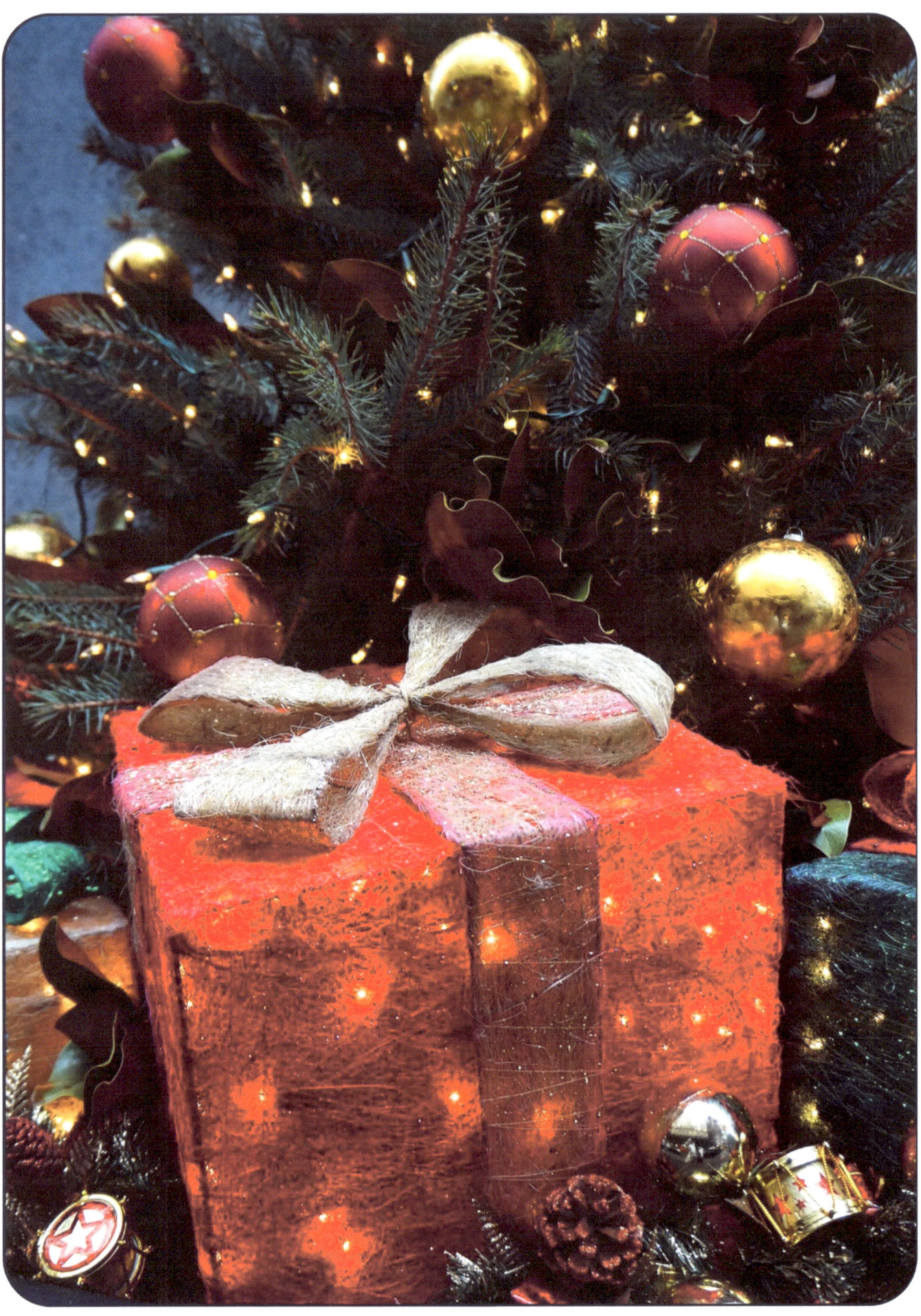

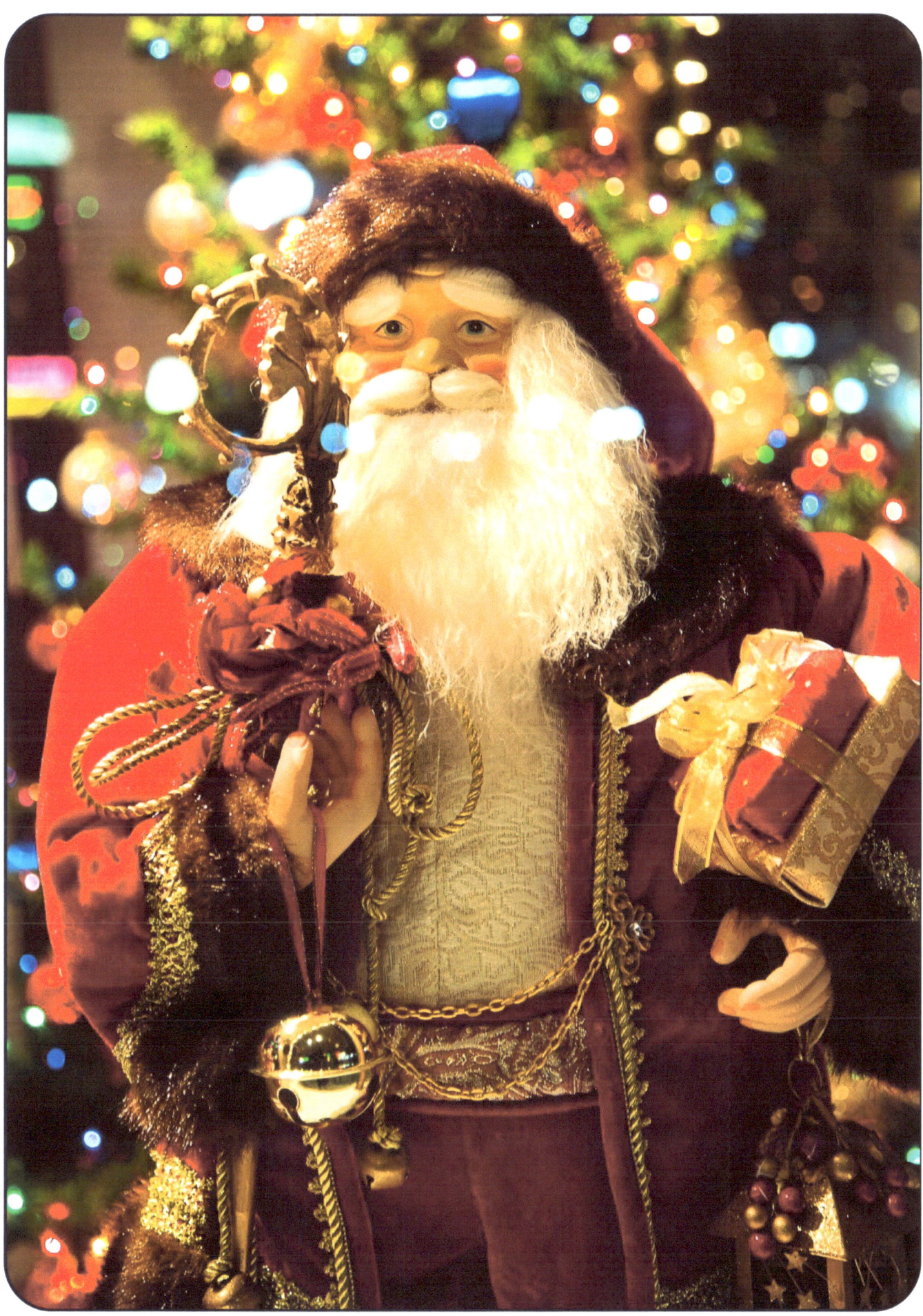

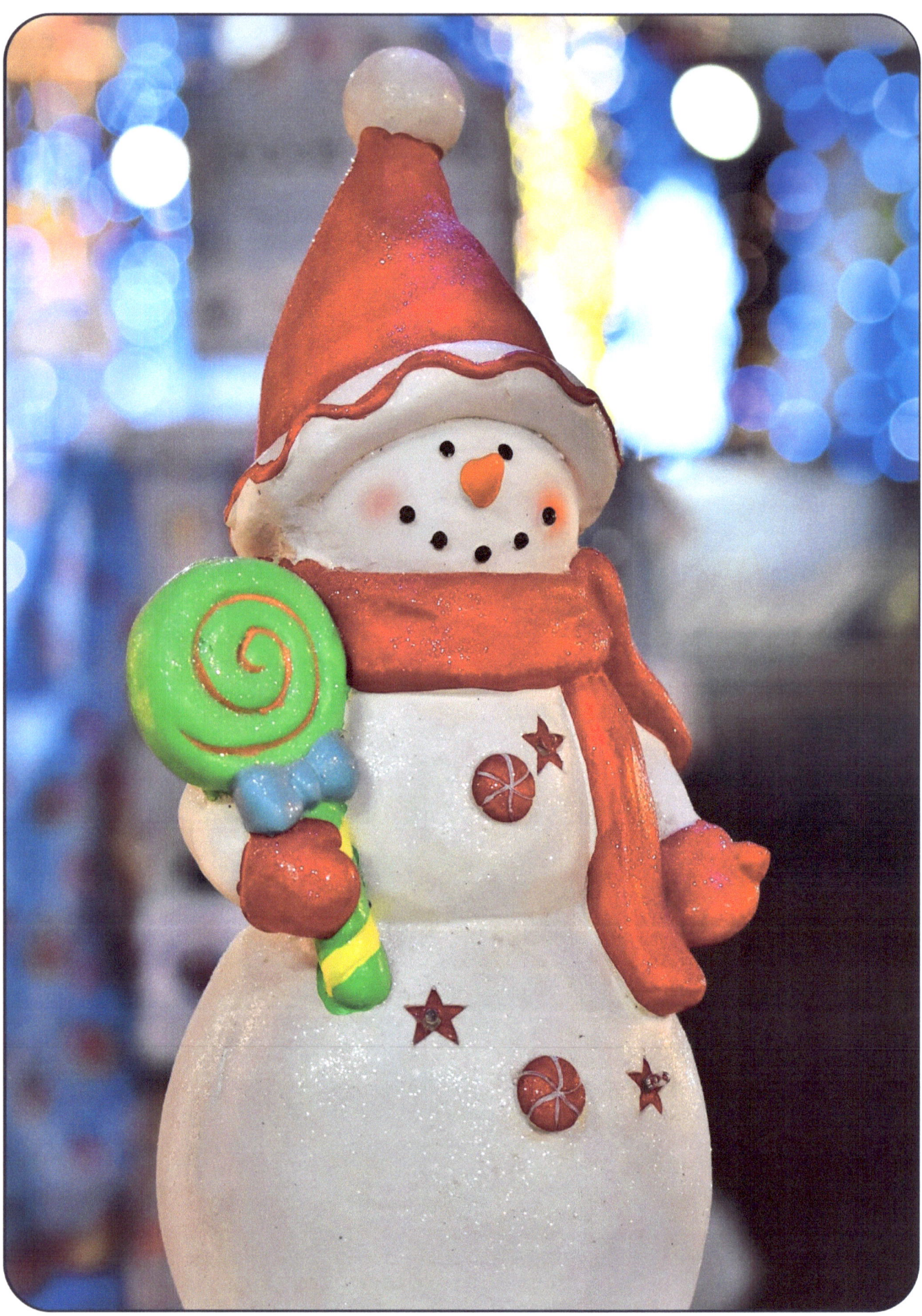

www.ingramcontent.com/pod-product-compliance
Lightning Source LLC
Chambersburg PA
CBHW041938240526
45473CB00037B/2203